EMERGING SYSTEMS IN LONG-TERM CARE

Paul R. Katz, MD
Robert L. Kane, MD
Mathy D. Mezey, RN, EdD, FAAN
Editors

Volume 4

 Springer Publishing Company

Copyright © 1999 by Springer Publishing Company, Inc.

All rights reserved

No part of this publication may be reproduced, stored in a retrieval system, or transmitted in any form or by any means, electronic, mechanical, photocopying, recording, or otherwise, without the prior permission of Springer Publishing Company, Inc.

Springer Publishing Company, Inc.
536 Broadway
New York, NY 10012-3955

Cover design by Janet Joachim
Acquisitions Editor: Helvi Gold
Production Editor: Jeanne Libby

01 02 03 / 5 4 3 2

ISBN: 0-8261-6835-3
ISSN: 1053-0606

Printed in the United States of America

Springer Series
ADVANCES IN LONG-TERM CARE

Series Editors: Paul R. Katz, MD
University of Rochester, School of Medicine and Dentistry

Robert L. Kane, MD
University of Minnesota, School of Public Health

Mathy D. Mezey, RN, EdD, FAAN
New York University, School of Nursing

Advisory Board: Laurence G. Branch, PhD, Elaine Brody, MSW, Alan M. Jette, PT, PhD, Rosalie A. Kane, DSW, Marshall B. Kapp, JD, MPH, Jurgis Karuza, PhD, Jeanie Kayser-Jones, RN, PhD, FAAN, M. Powell Lawton, PhD, John Morris, PhD, Joseph G. Ouslander, MD, Bruce C. Vladeck, PhD, William G. Weissert, PhD, Thelma Wells, RN, PhD, James G. Zimmer, MD

1991 Advances in Long-Term Care, Volume 1
P. R. Katz, MD, R. L. Kane, MD, M. D. Mezey, RN, EdD, FAAN

1993 Advances in Long-Term Care, Volume 2
P. R. Katz, MD, R. L. Kane, MD, M. D. Mezey, RN, EdD, FAAN

1995 Quality Care in Geriatric Settings: Focus on Ethical Issues
P. R. Katz, MD, R. L. Kane, MD, M. D. Mezey, RN, EdD, FAAN

1999 Emerging Systems in Long-Term Care
P. R. Katz, MD, R. L. Kane, MD, M. D. Mezey, RN, EdD, FAAN

Paul R. Katz, MD, is Associate Professor of Medicine at the University of Rochester School of Medicine and Dentistry. He is currently Medical Director at Monroe Community Hospital, Director of the Geriatric Fellowship Program at the University of Rochester, and Director of the Finger Lakes Geriatric Education Center. His research interests have focused on physician practice patterns in long-term care and organizational correlates of quality and medical education. He is co-editor of *Practice of Geriatrics, Principles and Practice of Nursing Home Care,* and *Psychiatric Care in the Nursing Home.* Dr. Katz is active in the American Geriatrics Society and the American Medical Director's Association and is involved in a number of national educational efforts.

Robert L. Kane, MD, was formerly the Dean of the University of Minnesota School of Public Health. He currently holds an endowed chair in Long-Term Care and Aging at the university and directs the University of Minnesota's Center on Aging and the Minnesota Area Geriatric Education Center. In addition, he also directs an NIA-funded training program in aging. Dr. Kane has conducted numerous research studies on both the clinical care and organization of care for older persons. The author of more than 20 books and 250 journal articles, Dr. Kane's recent publications in aging include the books *Essentials of Clinical Geriatrics* (Vol. 3) and *Heart of Long-Term Care.*

Mathy Doval Mezey, RN, EdD, FAAN, received her undergraduate and graduate education at Columbia University. She taught at Lehman College of the City University of New York. For 10 years she was a professor at the University of Pennsylvania School of Nursing where she directed the geriatric nurse practitioner program and was Director of the Robert Wood Johnson Foundation Teaching Nursing Home Program, a national initiative to link schools of nursing and nursing homes. Currently, Dr. Mezey is at New York University in the Division of Nursing where she holds a chair as the Independence Foundation Professor of Nursing Education and directs the Hartford Institute for Geriatric Nursing. Dr. Mezey has authored 5 books and has over 50 publications that focus on nursing care of the elderly and bioethical issues that affect decisions at the end of life. She is Series Editor for the Springer Series in Geriatric Nursing. Her current funded research and her writing focus on improving nursing care to older adults, and several studies that explore how best to improve decision making about life-sustaining treatment. Dr. Mezey is a Trustee of Columbia University, a Fellow in the Gerontological Society of America, and sits on the board of the Visiting Nurse Service of New York and the American Federation of Aging Research (AFAR).

Contents

Contributors		*vii*
Preface		*ix*
1	**Transitions Between Acute and Long-Term Care** *Mary D. Naylor and Paula Roe Prior*	1
2	**Subacute Care: Role and Implications for a Modernized Health Care System** *Steven A. Levenson*	23
3	**From Post-Acute to Chronic Care: Cost and Policy Implications of Medicare Home Health Expansion** *Penny Hollander Feldman*	45
4	**The Geriatric Day Hospital** *Lois K. Evans, Mary Ann Forciea, Johanna Yurkow, and Julie Sochalski*	67
5	**The PACE Model (Program for All Inclusive Care of the Elderly): A Review** *Paul Eleazer and Marsha Fretwell*	88
6	**Implications of Managed Care for Older Persons** *Robert Newcomer, Charlene Harrington, and Robert L. Kane*	118
7	**The "Voluntary" Status of Nursing Facility Admissions: Legal, Practice, and Public Policy Implications** *Marshall B. Kapp*	149
Index		*179*

Contributors

G. Paul Eleazer, MD, FACP
Division of Geriatrics
University of South Carolina School of Medicine
Columbia, SC

Lois K. Evans, DNSc, RN, FAAN
Professor and Director
Academic Nursing Practices
University of Pennsylvania School of Nursing
Philadelphia, PA

Penny Hollander Feldman, PhD
Director
Center for Home Care Policy and Research
Visiting Nurse Service of NY
New York, NY

Mary Ann Forciea, MD
University of Pennsylvania Schools of Nursing and Medicine
Philadelphia, PA

Marsha D. Fretwell, MD
Senior Care Systems PA
Clinical Associate Professor of Medicine
University of North Carolina at Chapel Hill
Chapel Hill, NC

Charlene Harrington, PhD
Department of Social and Behavioral Sciences
University of California
San Francisco, CA

Robert Kane, MD
Minnesota Chair in Long-Term Care and Aging
University of Minnesota School of Public Health
Minneapolis, MN

Marshall Kapp, JD, MPH
Professor, Community Health
Professor, Psychiatry
Director, Office of Geriatric Medicine and Gerontology
Wright State University
Dayton, OH

Steven Levenson, MD
Multi-facility Medical Director
Genesis ElderCare
Baltimore, MD

Mary Naylor, PhD, FAAN
Associate Dean
University of Pennsylvania School of Nursing
Philadelphia, PA

Robert Newcomer, PhD
Department of Social and Behavioral Sciences
University of California
San Francisco, CA

Paula Roe Prior, MSN
Doctoral Candidate
University of Pennsylvania School of Nursing
Philadelphia, PA

Julie Sochalski, PhD, RN, FAAN
University of Pennsylvania School of Nursing
Philadelphia, PA

Johanna Yurkow, MSN, CRNP
University of Pennsylvania School of Nursing
Philadelphia, PA

Preface

This volume, the fourth in a series, continues the tradition of exploring the intricacies and challenges inherent in long-term care. Over the past decade, the "Advances" series has spanned a broad array of topics ranging from epidemiologic predictions of future service needs to correlates of quality care by clinical site, the myths and realities of administrative law, to the policy and economic implications of new health care legislation.

Changes in health care continue at an unprecedented rate with long-term care receiving increasing attention. Such attention, in large part, is linked to the cost and processes of delivering care in the long-term care environment as well as the costs of chronic illness if not well managed. The issues broached in the pages that follow provide insight into these and related areas and highlight the dynamic nature of long-term care. As always, the authors of the current volume have been selected not only for their scholarly acumen but also because of the practical, real world insight that they possess.

In Chapter 1, Naylor and Prior begin by focusing on the critical transitions between acute and long-term care. Individuals in need of specific services as well as predictors of important clinical outcomes are explored in addition to current and emerging models of transitional care. Steve Levenson, in Chapter 2, describes the concept of subacute care from the systems perspective while detailing provider requirements and related reimbursement issues. In Chapter 3, Penny Feldman reviews the policy implications associated with the recent growth of Medicare home health services. Recognizing the vagaries of extant research, Dr. Feldman focuses on the potential for improving home care in an increasingly cost conscious environment. In Chapter 4, Lois Evans and colleagues review several community-based care models for older persons with a special focus on the development and overall effectiveness of the geriatric day hospital. Drs. Eleazer and Fretwell next present a review of the PACE model focusing on current evaluative and quality improvement efforts and cost-effectiveness as well as future directions for this innovative program. Drs. Newcomer, Harrington, and Kane continue in Chapter 6 by focusing on managed care and its implications for the burgeoning older population in need of long-term care services. Evidence is presented debunking myths surrounding managed care and traditional fee-for-service while the core elements of successful managed care programs and processes of care are highlighted. Finally, Chapter 7 explores the legal and ethical implications surrounding "involuntary" admissions to nursing homes. Marshall Kapp further unravels the vagaries of the nursing home admission process and its impact on accessibility for frail elders.

We hope that this volume will both inform and challenge the reader. While the vicissitudes of long-term care remain, the desire to better serve older people in need remains strong.

1
Transitions Between Acute and Long-Term Care

Mary D. Naylor
Paula Roe Prior

The recognition that acute care units in hospitals may not be the safest or most cost-effective site to provide patient care has led to the creation of new patient services. These services have been designed to serve as a bridge between acute care and patients' medical stability or between acute and long-term care. In the mid-1980s, the major impetus behind the establishment of alternatives to acute hospital care was Medicare's Prospective Payment System (PPS). More recently, the movement to managed care has stimulated development of these services. The term generally used to describe these alternatives is "transitional care." This chapter describes transitional care settings and explores issues related to their development; examines existing and emerging models of transitional care; and offers recommendations for future research.

TRANSITIONAL CARE SETTINGS: DESCRIPTIONS AND ISSUES

Transitional care is a broad term that encompasses a variety of settings including hospitals, home care agencies, nursing homes, rehabilitation centers, and patients' homes, and embraces a number of services including subacute, skilled, rehabilitative, and hospice. Commonly, transitional care refers to care and services that promote the safe and timely transfer of patients from one level of care to another (e.g., acute to subacute) or from one type of setting to another (e.g., hospital to home) (Brooten, 1993; Brooten & Naylor, in press). Transitional care, by definition, involves change—from illness to wellness, from dependence to self-care. Ideally, transitional care ends with a patient's recovery, functional or medical independence (Brooten, 1993; Brooten & Naylor, in press). For many frail elders, however, transitional care bridges the gap between acute and long-term care.

Changes in the delivery and financing of health care coupled with growing concerns about the solvency of the Medicare program have stimulated the development of a new health care industry known as transitional care (Aaron & Reischauer, 1995; Moon & Davis, 1995; Twentieth Century Fund, 1995). PPS has provided incentives for hospitals to create transitional care units so that patients could be moved from more costly beds and services. Earlier hospital discharge of more acutely ill elders resulted in a growing demand for Medicare-supported recuperative and rehabilitative services. The number of home health agencies, nursing homes, and rehabilitation centers has increased dramatically in response to this demand.

A number of studies have examined the use of transitional care services by Medicare beneficiaries since the introduction of PPS (Morrisey, Sloan, & Valrona, 1988; Neu & Harrison, 1988). Steiner and Neu (1992) found that the use of post-hospital care by a random sample of Medicare beneficiaries with short hospital stays varied by diagnosis-related groups (DRGs). Approximately 50% of patients with stroke, hip procedure, and hip fracture used some type of post-hospital care, while 25% of patients with heart disease and chronic obstructive pulmonary disease (COPD) used these services. Kane and colleagues (1996) found that almost 60% of the patients in their study of older adults discharged from 52 hospitals used post-acute care. There is great variation in the availability of different forms of transitional care across the country, especially certified rehabilitation units. Neu and Harrison (1988) have shown that nursing homes are sometimes used instead of rehabilitation centers, especially when the latter are in short supply. The continued development of transitional care services for older adults should be accompanied by research-based standards that help to identify the patients who would benefit most from these services; the nature and length of such services; the type and level of providers needed; and associated costs.

Patients in Need of Transitional Care Services

While older adults are recognized as a vulnerable population, not all require transitional care services. Naylor and colleagues (1994) demonstrated that many hospitalized elders who receive effective discharge planning do well after discharge. Research is helping to identify those patients who require transitional care services, with one group of studies focusing on factors contributing to poor post-discharge outcomes, while another is examining factors that influence the decision to refer to transitional care services.

Factors Related to Poor Outcomes

One way to approach the identification of patients in need of transitional care services is to examine the factors that contribute to poor outcomes for hospitalized elders. To date, research in this area has focused on predictors of hospital readmission, with particular attention paid to demographic and clinical variables (G. F. Anderson & Steinberg, 1984; Burns & Nichols, 1991; Reed, Pearlman, & Buchner, 1991; Vinson, Rich, Sperry, Shah, & McNamara, 1990).

Research findings regarding the influence of age are equivocal. Advancing age has been identified as the most consistent variable affecting the volume of service use (Alexander, Grumbach, Selby, Brown, & Washington, 1995; Bull, 1994; Corrigan & Martin, 1992; Mor, Wilcox, Rakowski, & Hiris, 1994). Elders, 85 and older, had a higher readmission rate after coronary artery bypass graft than did those under the age of 85 (Hennen, Krumholz, Radford, & Meehan, 1995). In other studies, however, age has not been found to be predictive of readmission for Medicare beneficiaries (Fethke, Smith, & Johnson, 1991; Reed et al., 1991; Vinson et al., 1990).

Males have been found to be at greater risk for rehospitalization (G. F. Anderson & Steinberg, 1984; Frank, Breeling, & Goldman, 1991). However, studies that have focused on patients with specific medical problems, such as heart failure, have not found gender to be predictive of readmission (Holloway, Thomas, & Shapiro, 1988; Vinson et al., 1990). While race and educational level have not been linked with hospital readmission (Ashton, Kuykendall, Johnson, Wray, & Wu, 1995), an annual income below $10,000 and/or eligibility for Medicaid have (G. F. Anderson & Steinberg, 1984; Weissman, Stern, & Epstein, 1994).

Clinical variables predictive of hospital readmission in older general medical patients include: a history of heart failure, diabetes mellitus, hypo- or hypertension; elevated white blood count; abnormal blood urea nitrogen or serum sodium levels; number of daily medications; and number of prior hospital admissions (Ashton et al., 1995; Burns & Nichols, 1991; Levine et al., 1996; Rich et al., 1995; Vinson et al., 1990). While surgical patients have a lower rehospitalization rate compared to medical patients, surgery in patients with a chronic medical condition such as heart disease, cancer and chronic obstructive pulmonary disease (COPD) increased the risk of readmission (Holloway et al., 1988). Disease-specific severity indices—composite clinical measures that are based on signs, symptoms and laboratory values—have also been found to be predictive of hospital readmission (Burns & Nichols, 1991; Reed et al., 1991).

In addition to demographic and clinical factors, there is evidence linking functional status, cognitive status, self-reported health status, social support, depression, and perceived quality of life to poor health outcomes among elders. Konstam and colleagues (1996) found that participants in the Left Ventricular Dysfunction clinical trials who reported poorer quality of life had increased readmissions for heart failure and increased mortality rates, even after controlling for a number of variables including age. Depression was found to predict readmission in older patients with heart disease (Levine et al., 1996). Using data from the Longitudinal Study on Aging, Mor and colleagues (1994) found that a less than excellent self-reported health score predicted disability, institutionalization and mortality, even after controlling for functional status and disease severity.

Often, a combination of factors have been linked to negative outcomes in older adults. Elders who rated their health as poor and had a chronic health problem such as heart failure or COPD were found to be at significantly higher risk for readmission (Holloway et al., 1988). Naylor and colleagues (1994) found that one or more of the following factors contributed to poor post-discharge outcomes among elders hospitalized with selected cardiac conditions: age 80 and older; inadequate or inaccessible support system; chronic problems requiring multiple medications/therapies; history of depression; moderate to severe functional impairment; hospitalization 30 days prior to index admission; multiple hospitalizations during 6 months prior to index admission; fair to poor self-rating of health; and history of nonadherence to therapeutic regimen.

Factors Influencing Clinical Decision Making

Another approach to identify patients in need of transitional care services is to examine the factors that influence clinical decision making related to referrals for these services. The decision to refer hospitalized elders for transitional care services is an integral part of a hospital's discharge planning process. This is a complex process often involving input from the patient, family, and many health team members. Currently, this process is highly influenced by Medicare's reimbursement requirements. For example, eligibility criteria for home health services after hospital discharge mandate that Medicare beneficiaries must be homebound; under the care of a physician; and in need of skilled nursing and/or physical, speech, or occupational therapy. Access to home health has not been influenced by differences in payment source including Medicare fee-for-service, Medicare HMO and dual Medicare-Medicaid enrollment (Experton, Branch, Ozminkowski, & Mellow-Lacey, 1997). There are, however, many other factors that influence clinicians' decisions to make referrals for transitional care services.

Referrals for transitional care services are often based on the patients' cognitive and functional abilities, availability of caregivers at home, ethnicity, geography, previous hospitalizations, and technology dependence (Corrigan & Martin, 1992; Gilmartin, 1994; Helberg, 1994; Prescott, Soeken, & Griggs, 1995). The decision that elders require discharge planning and follow-up services, for example, is often based on the patient's ability to perform activities of daily living (Branch et al., 1988; Cox, Wood, Montgomery, & Smith, 1990; Helberg, 1994; Kane et al., 1996; Kemper, 1992).

Unfortunately, there is no uniform method to evaluate a patient's functional ability during hospitalization. Reed and colleagues (1991) found that the only two measures of functional ability consistently recorded on patients' charts were orientation and ability to ambulate. Jones, Denson, and Brown (1989) discovered that 63% of elders with a deficit in one or more activity of daily living did not receive a referral for home services. Sixty percent of these patients reported that no one asked them how they would be able to manage their care after discharge.

Research findings suggest that clinicians can successfully identify those who do not need home care (non-need) but that there remains a group of patients in need of home care who are not identified (non-referred) (Prescott et al., 1995). In a convenience sample of 145 subjects, home care referrals were more common in patients who were older, had longer lengths of hospital stays, greater number of medical diagnoses, previous hospital admissions, higher levels of dependency and lower levels of physical functioning, social support, readiness for self-care and intent to adhere to treatment plan. Twenty-six percent of the sample, who were at a higher than average risk for poor outcomes, were not referred for home care. Other studies reinforce the finding that medical diagnosis is only one among a number of factors that may contribute to the need for care after hospital discharge. Numbers of comorbid conditions, number of medications, and use of therapies such as oxygen have also been linked to the need for home care after discharge (Narsavage, 1996).

Referrals to transitional services are also influenced by a patient's living situation (Kane et al., 1996). Living with someone frequently excludes the patient from receiving essential post-hospital services. Furstenberg and Mezey (1987) reported that 94% of patients who lived alone were visited by a discharge planner, while only 40% of those who lived with someone received such a visit. Using data generated from the Channeling demonstration project, Greene and Ondrich (1990) found that living alone increased the risk of nursing home placement while marital status did not. Kane and colleagues (1996) found that, for patients with a diagnosis of heart failure, the only significant predisposing factor predictive of both nursing home and home care referrals was living alone.

Pohl, Collins, and Given (1995) also found that access to transitional care services was influenced by sociodemographic characteristics. Blazer, Landerman, Fillenbaum, and Horner (1995) reported that being married made it more likely that an elder would have a usual health care provider and less likely that the elder would be hospitalized. Patients with a spouse as caregiver were less than half as likely to be referred for skilled nursing or home health aides when compared to those with non-spouse caregivers. Women with the same functional limitations as men were only about one-fourth as likely to be referred for home health services as men.

Geographic differences in the availability of services may result in a patient going without a needed service. Morris and Munasinghe's study (1994) examined the effect of geographic variability of hospital admission for Medicare patients with a diagnosis of COPD and discovered that the availability of hospital beds in an area had a positive association with hospital admission, while the number of physicians per capita had a negative impact on admission. Similarly, Fisher, Wennberg, Stukel, and Sharp (1994) found that significantly different readmission rates between two New England cities could not be accounted for by differences in severity of disease. The researchers postulated that having more available beds lowered the threshold for clinicians to readmit an elder.

The number and complexity of factors that may be predictive of hospital readmission and/or influence the decision to refer for transitional care support the need for risk screening instruments that could assist clinicians in the decision-making process. Solomon and colleagues (1993) proposed a model for predicting home care use after discharge. Four independent predictors were identified: Educational level < 12 years, less accessible social support, impairment in at least one instrumental activity of daily living (IADL), and prior home health care use. Additional variables that were found to be significant include female gender, ADL impairments, seven or more active medical diagnoses, and cognitive impairment.

Nature of Transitional Care Services, Providers, and Costs

Nature and Intensity of Transitional Care Services

In addition to early identification of elders in needs of these services, effective transitional care includes discharge planning, coordination and provision of appropriate services, and continued follow-up (Brooten, 1993). Shorter lengths of hospital stay and the increased demands on staff to address the needs of more acutely ill patients may result in staff having inadequate time to identify patients needing transitional services (Magilvy & Lakomy, 1991). These same factors may also affect the quality of discharge preparation that patients and caregivers receive. Several investigators have suggested a link between inadequate discharge preparation and unplanned hospital readmissions (Ghali, Kadakia, Cooper, & Ferlinz, 1988; Vinson et al., 1990).

Researchers have also suggested that the implementation of discharge plans may be a problem. Proctor et al. (1996) studied the extent to which discharge plans for older adults with congestive heart failure were implemented as planned. These investigators found that for 40% of patients, one or more components of the plan were not implemented as expected, resulting in unmet needs and less than adequate help and care. These discrepancies were more likely among low-income patients.

An important factor associated with effective discharge planning is the quality of communication among providers. A study of the adequacy of communication between hospital discharge planners and home health staff found that patient records contained only slightly more than half of the information needed to assure continuity of care (Anderson & Helms, 1993). Significantly more patient information was relayed to the home health staff when collected by a liaison nurse employed by the home care agency. Findings from this and other studies suggest that, even when discharge planning occurs, essential information may not be relayed to the providers of the next level of service. Poor communication may have a negative effect on patient outcomes (Harrington, Lynch, & Newcomer, 1993; Patterson, Leonard, & Titus, 1992).

Cloonan and Belyea (1993) examined 353 records of patients referred for skilled nursing after hospital discharge. In this study, functional impairments, cognitive impairment, medical diagnoses, age, length of hospital stay, and living alone were found to be related to the type and amount of home care received. Diwan, Berger, and Manns (1997) found that living alone increased the likelihood of receiving a homemaker, and that a decline in ADLs increased the odds of receiving a home health aide.

Race, culture, and ethnicity have been identified as factors influencing the nature of transitional care services used. Falcone, Bolda, and Leak (1991) reported that older Black patients were more likely to face a delay in hospital to nursing home placement than White patients, even after controlling for the complexity of care required and type of insurance coverage. Mui and Burnette (1994) reported that ethnicity was related to differences in the use of home care and community-based and nursing home services. White elders were more likely to use home care or nursing home services, while African-Americans and Hispanics tended to rely on informal support networks and community-based services. Kemper (1992) found race to be the only sociodemographic factor predictive of the amount or type of home care used, with African-Americans and Hispanics more likely than White patients to depend on informal care to meet their needs.

Other studies reinforce the influence of insurance (Freudenheim, 1996) and patient's distance from care sites (Kane et al., 1996). Even when a service is available locally, insurers may dictate that care be received at a distant site, or restrict access to certain providers and services (Fox, Wicks, & Newacheck, 1993; Harrington et al., 1993). After controlling for dependency and marital status, Morrow-Howell and Proctor (1994) found that being Medicaid-eligible or a private payer increased the likelihood that an elder would be discharged to a nursing home rather than to the home.

Kenney (1993) found that hospitals with swing beds, separate skilled nursing or intermediate care units, or both used less home health care, while hospitals with their own home care agencies discharged proportionately more patients to home health. In areas with more nursing home beds, there were fewer transfers to home care, while in states with more Medicaid skilled nursing beds, there were more Medicare beneficiaries discharged to home health. It is important to note that this study used data from 1985, only a few years after the introduction of PPS.

In summary, the nature of transitional care services is influenced by a number of factors, including quality of discharge planning, the needs of patients, the patient's living situation, race, culture, and ethnicity, geography, patient's insurance, and availability of services. Less well understood are the factors that influence the intensity of services that a patient receives.

Providers of Transitional Care Services

The providers of transitional care services are those clinicians and assistive personnel in the settings in which the care is provided. Although it is well recognized that many elders may require these services, there is disagreement about who should make decisions related to the nature and intensity of services needed, who should coordinate the care and, in some cases who should provide it (Kornowski, Zeeli, & Averbuch, 1995; Rich et al., 1995; Roselle & D'Amico, 1990; Schmitt, Farrell, & Heinemann, 1988).

The work of Brooten, Naylor, and colleagues (1986, 1988, 1994a, 1994b, 1995) using advanced practice nurses (APNs) to provide transitional care for high-risk patient groups has consistently demonstrated improved patient outcomes and health care savings for the patients studied. Advanced practice nurses have a master's degree in a specialty such as gerontological nursing and clinical expertise in the care of a selected patient population. The use of APNs has been tested primarily with the most vulnerable patient populations, ranging from very low birthweight infants and high-risk pregnant women to high-risk elders. The most appropriate provider(s) for lower-risk groups in need of transitional care services has not been reported.

The use of a multidisciplinary team to promote the successful transition of patients from one level of care to another has been advocated by many clinicians and scholars (Katz, 1993; Landefield, Palmer, Kresevic, Fortinsky, & Kowal, 1995; Rich et al., 1995; Wong, 1991). A multidisciplinary approach to guide discharge planning and follow-up is often needed by patients and families because of the complexity of health care needs. Schmitt et al. (1988) described a number of studies of team approaches to health care delivery for older adults, and discussed the challenging conceptual and methodological issues that investigators face in attempting to assess the effectiveness of interdisciplinary geriatric teams.

Costs for Transitional Care Services

Transitional care is often an episode of care across multiple settings, including discharge planning provided in a hospital, coordination of care between the hospital and the next level of care, and transitional services in the patient's home, a rehabilitation center or nursing home. Examining the costs of care delivered in one setting fails to capture the total costs of transitional services. There are, however, a number of challenges associated with collecting reliable and valid data across multiple settings. Studies that have attempted to measure these costs have generally not included indirect costs, such as the burden of care placed on families and the loss of employment, or benefits, such as the prevention of hospital readmissions or acute care visits to physicians. These data are important to understand the cost-benefit or cost-effectiveness of transitional care.

Current and Emerging Models of Transitional Care

Research-Based Models of Transitional Services

There are few examples of empirically based models of transitional care. An interdisciplinary model of transitional care delivered by APNs was developed by Brooten and colleagues in 1981 in response to national trends in earlier hospital discharge of vulnerable patient groups (Brooten et al., 1988). The Quality Cost Model of APN Transitional Care, developed for use with any vulnerable patient population, has undergone testing and refinement over the past two decades. This transitional care model, tested through a series of randomized clinical trials, has been demonstrated to improve quality and reduce health care costs across multiple, diverse patient groups (Brooten et al., 1986, 1994; Naylor et al., 1994; York et al., 1997).

The transitional services provided under this model are comprehensive discharge planning and home follow-up by APNs. The assumption underlying the use of APNs is that they have advanced knowledge and clinical skills in caring for the patient groups they follow and are prepared to deliver high quality, cost-effective care. The APN designs an individualized plan of care in collaboration with the patient, caregiver, patient's physicians, and other health team members. The same APN who designs the plan of care also implements it by providing direct clinical care in the home (substituting for the visiting nurses) and supervising and coordinating services provided by others.

The Day Hospital

The British health care system has long recognized the need for broad-based interdisciplinary care for older adults that facilitates transitions between and among homes, hospitals, and other health care settings. In response to this need, the system established the day hospital, an outpatient facility that provides intermittent care to community-dwelling older adults.

Although the research supporting this concept has been equivocal, only a few of the studies have examined day hospitals with a strong rehabilitation component. In a randomized trial conducted by Tucker, Davison, and Ogle (1984), elders cared for in a rehabilitative day hospital demonstrated significant improvement in the performance of ADLs 6 weeks after discharge, but not at the 5-month follow-up. The experimental group attended the day hospital 2 to 3 days a week for an average of 23 visits. The cost of the day hospital was one-third higher than usual care. Cummings and colleagues compared the effects of the day hospital versus inpatient rehabilitation services for elders on the use and cost of services and functional and physical health status (Cummings, Kerner, Arones, & Steinbock, 1985). Although the day hospital patients used more services, there was no difference between groups in physical and functional outcomes. The researchers hypothesized that the day hospital might be more cost-effective than inpatient care if the day setting maintained a high occupancy rate. No differences in functional status or quality of life were found in a randomized trial conducted by Eagle and colleagues (1991), who compared the outcomes of elders served in a rehabilitative day hospital versus usual care. A nurse-directed multidisciplinary team provided care at the day hospital for patients who attended twice a week. No cost data were reported.

Another example of a transitional care program based on the day hospital concept is the Collaborative Assessment and Rehabilitation for Elders (CARE) Program spearheaded by the School of Nursing at the University of Pennsylvania (Evans, Yurkow, & Siegler, 1995). This Gerontologic Nurse Practitioner (GNP)-managed interdisciplinary practice seeks to maximize functional status, promote health, and enhance the quality of life for frail elders. To qualify for the program, elders must meet the following admission criteria: Age over 65; need at least one rehabilitative service and one other service (i.e., psychiatry); be ineligible for inpatient rehabilitation; and be community-dwelling. Once admitted, elders undergo an extensive assessment by the GNP and a multidisciplinary team who design an individualized plan of care. Usually elders attend two to three half-day sessions a week for 2 to 9 weeks, depending on their assessed needs. Because the program has been certified as a Comprehensive Outpatient Rehabilitation Facility (CORF) it is eligible for Medicare and third-party reimbursement. Of the 21 patients who had completed the program by the spring of 1994, 71% had an improvement in functional status, and none showed a decline. These preliminary results support the feasibility and benefits of this GNP-directed intervention (Evans et al., 1995).

Home Health Care

Home health care is the fastest growing site for the delivery of transitional care services. Hospital-based and proprietary agencies have replaced public health agencies as the largest provider of this service as a result of Medicare changes in the late 1980s (National Association for Home Care [NAHC], 1995). Home care reimbursements grew from $2 billion in 1988 to $12.7 billion in 1994, accounting for more than 8% of the total Medicare budget (House Committee on Ways and Means, 1994). The explosive growth in home care is often attributed to the shorter length of hospital stays prompted by the PPS. However, a study conducted by Welch, Wennberg, and Welch (1996), using data from the 1993 Medicare National Claims History File, revealed that 78% of home health care visits occurred either longer than 1 month after a hospitalization, or were not associated with any inpatient care. Rather than acting as a transitional service, home care was being used primarily to provide long-term care, with more than half of the home care recipients receiving care for 6 months or more. Furthermore, findings from this study offered no evidence that services at home replace hospital services. There was wide geographic variation in the use of home health services, leading the authors to conclude that there exists a lack of consensus about the appropriate use of these services.

Community Nursing Services

Historically, visiting or public health nurses based in community agencies have coordinated and provided transitional care services. Their efforts have been supported by allied health professionals and home health aides. These nurses are familiar with the resources, values, and culture of the residents living in a community. Over the past two decades, significant budget reductions to these agencies have virtually eliminated services for many patient groups. Preventive health programs, for example, were curtailed or eliminated so that limited resources could be targeted to more acutely ill patients discharged earlier from hospitals (Bull, 1994; NAHC, 1995). As predicted by Moon and colleagues (1995), essential transitional services are now in jeopardy, as increased cuts imposed by the most recent budget reconciliation act threaten to decrease support for home follow-up of older adults.

One of the major challenges faced by these agencies has been to assure that staff are prepared to meet the increased acuity of patients discharged "quicker and sicker" from hospitals. Agencies are having to respond to these challenges at a time when insurers are providing decreased reimbursement (Brooten, 1995). Many have relied on APNs as consultants to address the continuing education needs of their staff (Zelle, 1995), while others with sufficient caseload have hired these expert clinicians to coordinate and/or deliver care to their high-risk patient groups.

Hospital-Based Home Care

Cost-containment efforts to substitute home care for more costly hospital stays have contributed to the growth of hospital-based home care. Hospitals have entered the home care field both to provide a safety net for patients and to generate revenues (Estes & Swan, 1994; Stahl, 1995). In most hospitals, home care services are provided by a staff hired and managed by the hospital's home care department (Brooten, 1995). One of the advantages of a hospital-based program is the internal availability of knowledgeable and skilled staff (Dahlberg & Koloroutis, 1994).

HMO Follow-up Services

Despite their initial reluctance, older adults are increasingly enrolling in HMOs, with both the federal government and business urging retirees into these plans (Butler & Moffitt, 1995; Wilensky, 1995). Similar to hospitals, HMOs have a clear incentive to discharge patients early. In addition, they have a special incentive to prevent hospital readmission. HMOs have used case managers including nurses and social workers to review patient's discharge and home care needs (Harrington et al., 1993; Retchin, Clement, Rossiter, Brown, & Nelson, 1992). More than the routine allowable number of home visits may be reimbursable for a patient, but this must be negotiated between the provider and insurer (Newcomer, Harrington, & Friedlob, 1990).

Sub-Acute Care

The sub-acute unit is an example of an innovative transitional care setting, one which has experienced rapid growth in the past decade (Stahl, 1994, 1995). These units are designed to meet the needs of medically stable patients who no longer require acute care services, but whose needs for licensed skilled nursing care exceed the abilities of skilled nursing facilities or nursing homes (Micheletti & Shlala, 1995; Stahl, 1994). Patients referred to subacute units include those who are technology-dependent, require frequent respiratory or physical therapy, or have complex nursing needs. To meet the needs of these patients, hospital beds are being converted to subacute beds, free standing subacute care hospitals are being established, and skilled nursing facilities are adding subacute units (Ellis & Mendlen, 1995; Micheletti & Shlala, 1995). Care is provided in a less expensive setting, hospital beds are freed up for acutely ill patients, and unoccupied beds are converted into a revenue source (Ellis & Mendlen, 1995; Stahl, 1994). In-hospital sub-acute care units have been reported to improve outcomes for selected patient populations, including older adults (Brymer et al., 1995; Landefield et al., 1995). The use of a multidisciplinary approach is believed to be a factor in the success of these units.

Some managed care organizations are contracting with nursing homes to provide elders with subacute care. Von Sternberg, Hepburn, Cibuzar, and Convey (1997) reported on a subacute care program developed for elders at a large Midwestern HMO in conjunction with five nursing homes. The HMO contracted with the sites to provide 15 beds for HMO members in need of subacute care. A higher nurse-to-patient ratio than was available in the rest of the facility was used. In return, the HMO provided the nursing home with board-certified geriatricians and geriatric nurse practitioners to work with the facilities' nurses, social workers, and therapists to meet the patients needs. When compared with elders served by nursing homes without this contract, elders in homes with this HMO contract had decreased lengths of nursing home stays and decreased per diem costs; hospital readmission rates were similar.

Integrated Health Systems

Managed care has stimulated the development of integrated health care delivery systems that are providing all levels of care including acute inpatient services, subacute care, home care, skilled nursing, ambulatory care, and durable medical supplies (Heller & Walston, 1995; Stahl, 1995). In theory, integrated systems provide continuity of care by having patients remain within the same delivery system (Stahl, 1995). In reality, fragmentation of care remains an issue, despite the use of case management and other approaches to coordinate care (Fox et al., 1993; Harrington et al., 1993).

Robinson, Mead, and Boswell (1995) described the efforts of one system to promote continuity of care across an acute care hospital, subacute unit, ambulatory service, nursing home, domiciliary unity, and extended day programs including adult day health. The system used hospital-based APNs to plan and coordinate patients' care across these settings. The APNs were also responsible for collaborating with other community agencies and nursing homes to which the patients were transferred. Communication among providers improved, resulting in less duplication of services; hospital admissions and lengths of stay also decreased.

Case Management

Although the case management model has been demonstrated to be a successful means to ensure continuity of care and coordination of services (Dorwart & Hoover, 1994; Robinson et al., 1995; Zelle, 1995) and many managed care organizations provide payment for primary care physician management, they do not always offer the comprehensive, multidisciplinary services required by many elders (Fox et al., 1993; Harrington et al., 1993). Even when a case manager is assigned to patients, their recommendations may not be relayed to or used by the patients' physicians (Harrington et al., 1993). Many authors have advocated a multidisciplinary, case management model to assure successful outcomes for patients requiring transitional care (Katz, 1993; Landefield et al., 1995; Rich et al., 1995; Wong, 1991).

Case management by nurses to coordinate the delivery of care to patients across settings may be an effective method of reducing fragmentation and improving patient and cost of care outcomes. One model of nurse case management was developed at Carondelet St. Mary's Hospital and Health Center to assist high-risk elders in managing their health care and accessing needed services in a timely and effective manner (Lamb, 1992). The nurse case manager is at the "hub" of the Nursing Network, the integrated system of nursing care at Carondelet St. Mary's (Ethridge & Lamb, 1989). Network components include acute inpatient care, extended care/long-term care, home care, and hospice and ambulatory care. Nurse case managers work with clients across settings and are responsible for facilitating the transition of patients throughout the Network. A study of the effects of this method of care revealed that elders who worked with a nurse case manager had greater confidence in self-care, improved symptom management, and less frequent use of hospital and emergency services (Lamb, 1992). This model of care also decreased hospital lengths of stay when compared to non-case managed patients (Ethridge & Lamb, 1989).

RECOMMENDATIONS FOR FUTURE RESEARCH

Transitional care environments are a relatively new dimension in the continuum of health care services. As a result, there are considerable gaps in knowledge to support this increasingly important component of care (Brooten & Naylor, in press). Additional research is needed to identify the profile of patients who would benefit most from these services and determine the nature and intensity of services needed to achieve positive patient and family outcomes, the type and level of providers needed to deliver these services, and the costs of services. Continued study of existing and emerging models of care is also necessary to identify which of these models achieve the highest-quality, most-effective outcomes.

Since transitional care has only recently been incorporated into the health care system, little research is available on the issue of access to services. As noted earlier, there is some evidence that race, ethnicity, economics, and geography are among the factors influencing access. Additional research is needed to understand the factors that either promote access or serve as barriers to transitional care.

Only a few of the approaches to transitional care are empirically based models. Research to date suggests that the core components of transitional care are comprehensive discharge planning and follow-up in homes, rehabilitation centers, and the like. Study findings also suggest that transitional care protocols designed to meet the unique needs of specific patient groups are more effective than the general discharge planning protocols used in most settings. Rigorous testing of transitional care protocols for many high-risk patient groups is needed to determine the efficacy of these protocols.

Research is needed to compare and contrast existing and emerging models of transitional services by examining both processes and outcomes achieved by these approaches. Knowledge generated from an examination of different models would inform the ongoing debate about which providers are most effective and efficient in providing continuity of care for patients and caregivers. These studies would also advance our understanding about effective ways to engage the perspectives of many disciplines in the design and implementation of transitional plans of care.

There are a number of methodological issues that need to be considered as part of a recommended agenda for transitional care; for example, what outcomes are important to examine, and when and for how long should they be measured. Transitional care provides a unique opportunity to explore the contributions of different health care providers and family members because of the nature and length of service.

In summary, transitional care is emerging as a critical component of the U.S. health care system. At the same time, cuts in Medicare are threatening access of elders to these services. Additional research is essential to increase the knowledge base to identify the needs of patients and caregivers during the critical periods of transition. Research will also assist in determining the most effective and efficient models for the growing population of older adults.

REFERENCES

Aaron, H. J., & Reischauer, R. D. (1995). The Medicare reform debate: What is the next step? *Health Affairs, 14,* 8–30.

Alexander, M., Grumbach, K., Selby, J., Brown, A., & Washington, E. (1995). Hospitalization for congestive heart failure. *Journal of the American Medical Society, 274,* 1037–1042.

Anderson, G. F., & Steinberg, E. P. (1984). Hospital readmissions in Medicare population. *The New England Journal of Medicine, 311,* 1349–1353.

Anderson, M. A., & Helms, L. (1993). An assessment of discharge planning models: Communication in referrals to home care. *Orthopedic Nursing, 12,* 41–49.

Ashton, C. M., Kuykendall, D. H., Johnson, M. L., Wray, N. P., & Wu, L. (1995). The association between the quality of inpatient care and early admission. *Annals of Internal Medicine, 122,* 415–421.

Blazer, D. G., Landerman, L. R., Fillenbaum, G., & Horner, R. (1995). Health services access and use among older adults in North Carolina: Urban vs rural residents. *American Journal of Public Health, 85,* 1384–1390.

Branch, L. G., Wetle, T. T., Scherr, P. A., Cook, N. R., Evans, D. A., Hebert, L. E., Masland, E. N., Keough, M. E., & Taylor, J. O. (1988). A prospective study of incident comprehensive medical home care use among the elderly. *The American Journal of Public Health, 78,* 255–259.

Brooten, D. (1993). Assisting with transitions from hospital to home. In S. Funk, E. Tornquist, M. Champagne, & R. Wiese (Eds.), *Key aspects of caring for the chronically ill: Hospital and home.* New York: Springer Publishing Co.

Brooten, D., Brown, L., Munro, B., York, R., Cohen, S., Roncoli, M., & Hollingsworth, A. (1988). Early discharge and specialist transitional care. *Image: The Journal of Nursing Scholarship, 20,* 64–68.

Brooten, D., Kumar, S., Brown, L., Butts, P., Finkler, S., Bakewell-Sachs, S., Gibbons, A., & Delivoria-Papadapoulos, M. (1986). A randomized clinical trial of early discharge and home follow-up of very low birthweight infants. *The New England Journal of Medicine, 315,* 934–939.

Brooten, D., & Naylor, M. (in press). Transitional environments that optimize outcomes. In A. S. Hinshaw, S. Feetham, & J. Shaver (Eds.), *Handbook of clinical nursing research.* Thousand Oaks, CA: Sage.

Brooten, D., Naylor, M., York, R., Brown, L., Roncoli, M., Hollingsworth, A., Cohen, S., Arnold, L., Finkler, S., Munro, B., & Jacobsen, B. (1995). Effects of nurse specialist transitional care on patient outcomes and cost: Results of five randomized trials. *The American Journal of Managed Care, 1,* 35–41.

Brooten, D., Roncoli, M., Finkler, S., Arnold, L., Cohen, A., & Mennuti, M. (1994). A randomized clinical trial of early hospital discharge and home follow-up of women having cesarean birth. *Obstetrics and Gynecology, 84,* 832–838.

Brymer, C. D., Kohm, C. A., Naglie, G., Shekter-Wolfson, L., Zorzitto, M. L., O'Rourke, K., & Kirkland, J. L. (1995). Do geriatric programs decrease long-term use of acute care beds? *Journal of the American Geriatrics Society, 43,* 885–889.

Bull, M. J. (1994). Use of formal community services by elders and their family caregivers 2 weeks following hospital discharge. *Journal of Advanced Nursing, 19,* 503–508.

Burns, R. B., McCarthy, E. P., Moskowitz, M. A., Ash, A., Kane, R. L., & Finch, M. (1997). Outcomes for older men and women with congestive heart failure. *Journal of the American Geriatrics Society, 45,* 276–280.

Butler, S. M., & Moffitt, R. E. (1995). The FEAS as a model for a new Medicare Program. *Health Affairs, 14,* 47–60.

Cloonan, P. A., & Belyea, M. J. (1993). Limits of using patient characteristics in predicting home health care coordination. *Western Journal of Nursing Research, 15,* 742–751.

Corrigan, J. M., & Martin, J. B. (1992). Identification of factors associated with hospital readmission and development of a predictive model. *Health Services Research, 27,* 81–101.

Cox, C. L., Wood, J. E., Montgomery, A. C., & Smith, P. C. (1990). Patient classification in home health care: Are we ready? *Public Health Nursing, 7,* 130–137.

Cummings, V., Kerner, J. F., Arones, S., & Steinbock, C. (1985). Day hospital service in rehabilitation medicine: An evaluation. *Archives of Physical Medical Rehabilitation, 66,* 86–91.

Dahlberg, N. L., & Koloroutis, M. (1994). Hospital-based perinatal home-care program. *Journal of Obstetric, Gynecologic, and Neonatal Nursing, 23,* 682–686.

Diwan, S., Berger, C., & Manns, E. K. (1997). Composition of the home care service package: Predictors of type, volume, and mix of services provided to poor and frail older people. *The Gerontologist, 37,* 169–181.

Dorwart, R. A., & Hoover, C. W. (1994). A national study of transitional hospital services in mental health. *American Journal of Public Health, 84,* 1229–1234.

Eagle, D. J., Guyatt, G. H., Patterson, C., Turpie, I., Sackett, B., & Singer, J. (1991). Effectiveness of a geriatric day hospital. *Canadian Medical Association Journal, 144,* 699–704.

Ellis, S., & Mendlen, J. (1995). Teaming up with hospitals. *Provider, 21,* 35–36.

Estes, C. L., & Swan, J. H. (1994). Privatization, system membership, and access to home health care for the elderly. *The Milbank Quarterly, 72,* 277–298.

Etheridge, P., & Lamb, G. S. (1989). Professional nursing case management improves quality, access and costs. *Nursing Management, 20,* 30–35.

Experton, B., Li, Z., Branch, L. G., Ozminkowski, R. J., & Mellow-Lacey, D. M. (1997). The impact of payor/provider type on health care use and expenditures among the frail elderly. *American Journal of Public Health, 87*(2), 210–216.

Evans, L. K., Yurkow, J., & Siegler, E. L. (1995). The CARE Program: A nurse-managed collaborative outpatient program to improve function of frail older people. *Journal of the American Geriatrics Society, 43,* 1155–1160.

Falcone, D., Bolda, E., & Leak, S. C. (1991). Waiting for placement: An exploratory analysis of determinants of delayed discharges of elderly hospital patients. *Health Services Research, 26,* 339–374.

Fethke, C. C., Smith, I. M., & Johnson, N. (1991). Risk factors affecting readmission of the elderly into the health care system. *Medical Care, 24,* 429–437.

Fisher, E. S., Wennberg, J. E., Stukel, T. A., & Sharp, S. M. (1994). Hospital readmission rates for cohorts of Medicare beneficiaries in Boston and New Haven. *The New England Journal of Medicine, 331,* 989–995.

Fox, H. B., Wicks, L. B., & Newacheck, P. W. (1993). Health maintenance organizations and children with special needs: A suitable match? *American Journal of the Disabled Child, 147,* 546–552.

Frankl, S. E., Breeling, J. L., & Goldman, L. (1991). Preventability of emergent hospital readmission. *The American Journal of Medicine, 90,* 667–674.

Freudenheim, M. (1996, April 29). A.A.R.P. will license its name to managed health care plans. *The New York Times.*

Furstenberg, A. L., & Mezey, M. D. (1987). Mental impairment of elderly hospitalized hip fracture patients. *Comprehensive Gerontology, 1,* 80–85.

Ghali, K., Kadakia, S., Cooper, R., & Ferlinz, J. (1988). Precipitating factors leading to decompensation of heart failure. *Archives of Internal Medicine, 148,* 2013–2016.
Gilmartin, M. (1994). Transition from the Intensive Care Unit to home: Patient selection and discharge planning. *Respiratory Care, 39,* 456–480.
Greene, V. L., & Ondrich, J. I. (1990). Risk factors for nursing home admissions and exits: A discrete-time hazard function approach. *Journal of Gerontology, 45,* S250–S258.
Harrington, C., Lynch, M., & Newcomer, R. J. (1993). Medical services in social health maintenance organizations. *The Gerontologist, 33,* 790–800.
Helberg, J. L. (1994). Use of home care nursing resources by the elderly. *Public Health Nursing, 11,* 104–112.
Heller, J. F., & Walton, J. R. (1995). The postacute link. *RT: The Journal for Respiratory Care Practitioners, 8,* 153–155.
Hennen, J., Krumholz, H. M., Radford, M. J., & Meehan, T. P. (1995). Readmission rates, 30 days and 365 days postdischarge, among the 20 most frequent DRG groups, Medicare inpatients age 65 or older in Connecticut hospitals, fiscal years 1991, 1992, and 1993. *Connecticut Medicine, 59,* 263–270.
Holloway, J. J., Thomas, J. W., & Shapiro, L. (1988). Clinical and sociodemographic risk factors for readmission of Medicare beneficiaries. *Health Care Financing Review, 10,* 27–36.
House Committee on Ways and Means. (1994). *Overview of entitlement programs* (Publication Number: WMCP:103-27). Washington, DC: Government Printing Office.
Jones, E. W., Densen, P. M., & Brown, S. D. (1989). Posthospital needs of elderly people at home: Findings from an eight-month follow-up study. *Health Services Research, 24,* 643–664.
Kane, R. L., Finch, M., Blewett, L., Chen, Q., Burns, R., & Moskowitz, M. (1996). Use of post-hospital care by Medicare patients. *Journal of the American Geriatrics Society, 44,* 242–250.
Katz, K. S. (1993). Project Headed Home: Intervention in the Pediatric Intensive Care Unit for infants and their families. *Infants & Young Children, 5,* 67–75.
Kemper, P. (1992). The use of formal and informal home care by the disabled elderly. *Health Services Research, 27,* 421–451.
Kenney, G. M. (1993). How access to long-term care affects home health transfers. *Journal of Health Politics, Policy, and Law, 18,* 937–965.
Konstam, V., Salem, D., Pouleur, H., Kostis, J., Gorkin, L., Shumaker, S., Mottard, I., Woodes, P., Konstam, M. A., & Yusuf, S. (1996). Baseline quality of life as a predictor of mortality and hospitalization in 5,025 patients with congestive heart failure. *American Journal of Cardiology, 78,* 890–895.
Kornowski, R., Zeeli, D., & Averbuch, M. (1995). Intensive home-care surveillance prevents hospitalization and improves morbidity rates among elderly patients with severe congestive heart failure. *American Heart Journal, 129,* 762–766.
Lamb, G. (1992). *Conceptual and methodological issues in nurse case management research.* Washington, DC: American Nurses' Publishing.

Landefield, C. S., Palmer, R. M., Kresevic, D. M., Fortinsky, R., & Kowal, J. (1995). A randomized trial of care in hospital medical unit especially designed to improve the functional outcomes of acutely ill older patients. *New England Journal of Medicine, 32,* 1333–1338.

Levine, J. B., Covino, N. A., Slack, W. V., Safran, C., Safran, D. B., Boro, J. E., Davis, R. B., Buchanan, G. M., & Gervino, E. V. (1996). Psychological predictors of subsequent medical care among patients hospitalized with cardiac disease. *The Journal of Cardiopulmonary Rehabilitation, 16,* 109–116.

Magilvy, J. K., & Lakomy, J. M. (1991). Transitions of older adults to home care. *Home Health Care Services Quarterly, 12,* 59–70.

Micheletti, J. A., & Shlala, T. J. (1995). Understanding and operationalizing subacute services. *Nursing Management, 26,* 51–52, 54–56.

Moon, M., & Davis, K. (1995). Preserving and strengthening Medicare. *Health Affairs, 14,* 31–46.

Mor, V., Wilcox, V., Rakowski, W., & Hiris, J. (1994). Functional transitions among the elderly: Patterns, predictors, and related hospital use. *American Journal of Public Health, 84,* 1274–1280.

Morris, R. D., & Munasinghe, R. L. (1994). Geographic variability in hospital admission rates for respiratory disease among the elderly in the United States. *Chest, 106,* 1172–1181.

Morrisey, M. A., Sloan, F. A., & Valvona, J. (1988). Shifting Medicare patients out of the hospital. *Health Affairs, 7,* 52–64.

Morrow-Howell, N., & Proctor, E. (1994). Discharge destinations of Medicare patients receiving discharge planning: Who goes where? *Medical Care, 32,* 486–497.

Mui, A. C., & Burnette, D. (1994). Long-term care service use by frail elders: Is ethnicity a factor? *The Gerontologist, 34,* 190–198.

Narsavage, G. L. (1996). The influence of symptoms, lung function, mood, and social support on the level of functioning patients with COPD. *Perspectives in Respiratory Nursing, 7,* 6–7.

National Association for Home Care. (1995). *Basic statistics about home care 1995.* Washington, DC: Author.

Naylor, M., Brooten, D., Jones, R., Lavizzo-Mourey, R., Mezey, M., & Pauly, M. (1994). Comprehensive discharge planning for the hospitalized elderly. *Annals of Internal Medicine, 120,* 999–1006.

Neu, C. R., & Harrison, S. C. (1988). *Posthospital care before and after the Medicare prospective payment system.* Santa Monica, CA: Rand.

Newcomer, R., Harrington, C., & Friedlob, A. (1990). Social health maintenance organizations. *Gerontologist, 30,* 86–93.

Patterson, J. M., Leonard, B. J., & Titus, J. C. (1992). Home care for medically fragile children: Impact on family health and well-being. *Developmental & Behavioral Pediatrics, 13,* 248–255.

Pohl, J. M., Collins, C., & Given, C. W. (1995). Beyond patient dependency: Family characteristics and access of elderly patients to home care services following hospital discharge. *Home Health Care Services Quarterly, 15,* 33–47.

Prescott, P. A., Soeken, K. L., & Griggs, M. (1995). Identification and referral of hospitalized patients in need of home care. *Research in Nursing and Health, 18,* 85–95.

Proctor, E. K., Morrow-Howell, N., & Kaplan, S. J. (1996). Implementation of discharge plans for chronically ill elders discharged home. *Health and Social Work, 21,* 30–40.

Reed, R. L., Pearlman, R. A., & Buchner, D. M. (1991). Risk factors for early unplanned hospital readmission in the elderly. *Journal of General Internal Medicine, 6,* 223–228.

Retchin, S. M., Clement, D. G., Rossiter, L. F., Brown, B., & Nelson, L. (1992). How the elderly fare in HMOs: Outcomes from the Medicare Competition Demonstrations. *Health Services Research, 27,* 651–669.

Rich, M. W., Beckham, V., Wittenberg, C., Leven, C. L., Freedland, K. E., & Carney, R. M. (1995). A multidisciplinary intervention to prevent the readmission of elderly patients with congestive heart failure. *The New England Journal of Medicine, 333,* 1190–1195.

Robinson, D. K., Mead, M. J., & Boswell, C. R. (1995). Inside looking out: Innovations in community health nursing. *Clinical Nurse Specialist, 9,* 227–229, 235.

Roselle, S., & D'Amico, F. J. (1990). The effect of home respiratory therapy on hospital readmission rates of patients with chronic obstructive pulmonary disease. *Respiratory Care, 35,* 1208–1213.

Schmitt, M. H., Farrell, M. P., & Heinemann, G. D. (1988). Conceptual and methodological problems in studying the effects of interdisciplinary geriatric teams. *The Gerontologist, 28,* 753–764.

Solomon, D. H., Wagner, D. R., Marenberg, M. E., Acampora, D., Cooney, L. M., & Inouye, S. K. (1993). Predictors of formal home health care use in elderly patients after hospitalization. *Journal of the American Geriatric Society, 41,* 961–966.

Stahl, D. (1994). Subacute care: The future of health care. *Nursing Management, 25,* 34–40.

Stahl, D. (1995). The changing managed care arena: Impact on subacute care. *Nursing Management, 26,* 16–17.

Steiner, A., & Neu, C. R. (1992). *Monitoring the changes in use of Medicare posthospital services.* Santa Monica, CA: Rand.

Tucker, M. A., Davison, J. G., & Ogle, S. J. (1984). Day hospital rehabilitation. Effectiveness and cost in the elderly: A randomized controlled trial. *British Medical Journal, 298,* 1209–1212.

Twentieth Century Fund. (1995). *Medicare reform: A Twentieth Century Fund guide to the issues.* New York: Twentieth Century Fund Press [http//epn.org/tcf/tcmedi.html]

Vinson, J. M., Rich, M. W., Sperry, C., Shah, A. S., & McNamara, T. (1990). Early readmission of elderly patients with congestive heart failure. *Journal of the American Geriatric Society, 38,* 1290–1295.

Von Sternberg, T., Hepburn, K., Cibuzar, P., & Convey, L. (1997). Post-hospital sub-acute care: An example of a managed care model. *Journal of the American Geriatrics Society, 45,* 87–91.

Weissman, J. S., Stern, R. S., & Epstein, A. M. (1994). The impact of patient socioeconomic status and other social factors on readmission: A prospective study in four Massachusetts hospitals. *Inquiry, 31,* 163–172.

Welch, H. G., Wennberg, D. E., & Welch, W. P. (1996). The use of Medicare home health care services. *New England Journal of Medicine, 335,* 324–329.

Wilensky, G. R. (1995). The score on Medicare reform: Minus the hype and hyperbole. *The New England Journal of Medicine, 333,* 1774–1777.

Wong, D. L. (1991). Transition from hospital to home for children with complex medical care. *Journal of Pediatric Oncology Nursing, 8,* 3–9.

York, R., Brown, L. P., Samuels, P., Finkler, S. A., Jacobsen, B., Persely, C. A., Swank, A., & Robbin, D. (1997). A randomized trial of early discharge and nurse specialist transitional follow-up care of high-risk childbearing women. *Nursing Research, 46,* 254–261.

Zelle, R. S. (1995). Follow-up of at-risk infants in the home setting: Consultation model. *Journal of Obstetrical, Gynecological and Neonatal Nursing, 24,* 51–55.

2
Subacute Care: Role and Implications for a Modernized Health Care System

Steven A. Levenson

Subacute care is not a new service, but it has become more widespread in various settings. Subacute programs care for individuals in various stages of acute illness and injury, usually after—but sometimes instead of—hospitalization for an acute episode. This article presents an update on the conceptual, clinical, regulatory, and reimbursement aspects of subacute care.

FACTORS PROMOTING GROWTH OF SUBACUTE CARE

Subacute care is not new, although the widespread use of the term "subacute" has arisen only in the past few years. Three decades ago, Federal Medicare programs established a Skilled Nursing Facility category for providing post-acute care. Other sites that have been providing such care for several decades include long-term or "chronic care" hospitals, extended care facilities, and specialty hospitals.

Several factors have stimulated the growth of subacute care in the 1990s. These include a growing aged population, an increase in survivors of serious illnesses and injuries, and advances in medical knowledge and technology enabling more sophisticated treatments to be delivered in non-hospital settings. However, economics has been the primary driver of subacute care. In particular, concern over the high costs of hospitalization has prompted the search for alternative settings and programs.

SHIFTS IN SETTINGS FOR HEALTH CARE DELIVERY

Service delivery is often no longer strictly associated with a discrete care site. The term "subacute care" is better used to describe a program than a specific site. This reflects a general shift within the health care delivery system. Until recently, health care delivery sites were typically associated with discrete levels of care and services. Acute hospitals treated serious acute illness and injury; nursing homes and other similar facilities gave long-term care to those with serious chronic disabilities; and less serious care needs were met through combinations of ambulatory and home-based care.

However, these distinctions are increasingly less relevant, as health care is now being delivered throughout a continuum of care sites. Various levels of care are now given at the same site, and different sites now deliver similar levels of care. For example, more than half of all surgery in the U.S. is performed on an outpatient basis, and a spectrum of rehabilitation services is being provided in every setting from homes to hospitals.

Acute care hospitals increasingly specialize primarily as sites for the short-term evaluation and management of complicated or life-threatening acute conditions. They tend to focus on identifying and initiating management of the causes of acute illness and injury than on addressing the consequences. They are no longer expected to handle the full spectrum of patient needs or the entire span of their acute illnesses. Other settings and practitioners are increasingly able to manage uncomplicated acute illnesses and the later stages of more complex conditions, including the continuing treatment of partially resolved conditions, management of other coexisting problems and illnesses, delivery of rehabilitative and restorative care, and handling of the longer-range ethical and psychosocial consequences of illness.

THE VARIOUS FACETS OF ILLNESS AND INJURY

Medical illness has various aspects and influences. It is important to identify and understand these, in order to understand the variety of subacute care that is offered.

An acute illness may be defined as a rapid or sudden onset of a detectable alteration in bodily structure or function. An injury is a significant disruption of bodily structure or function as a result of some external physical contact (a fall, auto accident, medical treatment, etc.) or the introduction of an external substance (medication, radiation, poison, etc.) into the body.

Minor or self-limited acute illnesses (upper respiratory infections, viral gastroenteritis, etc.) or injuries (minor sprains, contusions, etc.) require little or no professional care. Other illnesses and injuries cause individuals to need some help. Possible outcomes of an acute problem may be for full or partial improvement, stabilization (prevention of further decline), decline, or death. Illnesses may also cause or be influenced by other physical, functional, and psychosocial problems (Table 2.1).

Factors Influencing Outcomes of Episodes of Illness and Injury

Medical illness has various aspects and influences. Outcomes appear to be consistently influenced by three categories of factors: acuity (severity

TABLE 2.1 Various Consequences and Complications of Acute Illness

Situation	Example
Acute condition and consequences both resolve fully	• Respiratory distress and functional deficits resolve when pneumonia resolves • Impaired mobility resolves when pelvic fracture heals
Acute condition resolves fully, but some consequences remain	• Stroke patient has residual speech deficit and left-sided weakness long after stroke has stabilized
Acute condition resolves, but underlying conditions remain	• Despite curing an infection, an AIDS patient continues to suffer other complications
Acute condition resolves, but it aggravates other coexisting conditions	• Episode of acute congestive heart failure improves but leaves a mildly demented individual weaker and more confused
Acute condition improves partially, but individual still needs prolonged treatment to enable fuller resolution	• Endocarditis or osteomyelitis patients need lengthy antibiotic therapy • Ventilatory failure patients may be stabilized quickly, but some may need months of care before being able to breathe without ventilatory assistance

of illness), comorbidity, and function. A discrete number of factors found to influence patient outcomes may be categorized as physical, functional, or psychosocial factors reflecting severity of illness, comorbidity, functional dependency, or some combination of these (Table 2.2) (Ceder, Thorngren, & Walden, 1980; Cleves, Sanchez, & Draheim, 1997; Greenfield, Apolone, McNeil, & Cleary, 1993; Jette, Harris, Clearly, & Campion, 1987; Levenson, 1996; Magaziner, Simonick, Kashner, Hebel, & Kenzora, 1990; Muder, Brennen, Swensen, & Wagener, 1996; Newschaffer, Bush, & Penberthy, 1997; O'Keefe & Lavan, 1997; Poses, McClish, Smith, Bekes, & Scott, 1996; Rochon et al., 1996; Zureik et al., 1997).

CHARACTERIZING SUBACUTE CARE

Subacute patients may have various primary acute problems (Table 2.3). However, patients' admitting diagnosis or principal treatment or service may not fully reflect the scope of their relevant problems. Rehabilitation (Parmelee, Thuras, Katz, & Lawton, 1995) and psychiatric (Bernardini,

TABLE 2.2 Summary of Relevant Patient-Related Factors Influencing or Predicting Outcomes (As Published in Diverse Medical Literature)

Physical
- Severity of illness
- Comorbidities (number/severity)
- Nutritional status/Weight loss
- Depression
- Delirium
- "General deconditioning"
- Presence of infection
- Diseases: neurological, cardiac, cancer; diabetes

Functional
- Impaired baseline ADL status
- Number of ADL dependencies
- Weighted ADL dependency score
- Self-reported limitations on physical functioning
- Hearing loss
- Gait velocity, balance function, and grip strength

Psychosocial
- Discharge to a place other than home
- Level of family support and interest

TABLE 2.3 Typical Primary Reasons for Hospitalization Prior to a Subacute Stay

- Pelvic fracture
- Syncope/falling/orthostatic hypotension
- Weakness/lethargy
- Acute confusion
- Auto accident
- Chronic Obstructive Pulmonary Disease (COPD) exacerbation
- Acute myocardial infarction
- Metastatic breast and colon carcinoma
- Urinary tract infection
- Pneumonia
- Skin ulcers
- Cellulitis
- Infectious arthritis
- Gangrenous foot
- Pancreatitis
- Dehydration

Meinecke, Pagani, Grillo, Fabbrini, Zaccarini, Corsini, Scapellato, & Bonaccorso, 1995) patients often have underlying medical problems or complications. Medical patients have functional and psychosocial needs (Incalzi, Capparella, Gemma, Porcedda, Raccis, Sommella, & Carbonin, 1992; Moos & Mertens, 1996).

Many acutely ill or injured patients have various comorbidities (Table 2.4). *Comorbidities* (or coexisting conditions) may represent a complication of an acute illness (for example, a lung abscess complicating pneumonia); a pre-existing condition that was present when the acute illness began (for example, rheumatoid arthritis or hypertension); a risk factor that could

TABLE 2.4 Typical Comorbidities of Subacute Patients

- COPD
- Hypertension
- Diabetes mellitus
- Arteriosclerotic cardiovascular disease
- Congestive heart failure
- Cardiac arrhythmias
- Osteoporosis
- Dementia

exacerbate a current illness (for example, a Foley catheter placed in a post-operative hip replacement patient creates a risk factor for a systemic urinary tract infection, which could lead to death); or a new condition that arises or is first detected at the time of an acute illness but is not necessarily related to that illness (for example, a patient with a new myocardial infarction is found to have diabetes).

Acuity or "severity of illness" represents the overall intensity or impact of an episode of illness. This burden is influenced by physiological elements and by functional and psychosocial factors (Rosenthal, Halloran, Kiley, Pinkley, & Landefeld, 1995; Satish, Winograd, Chavez, & Bloch, 1996). *Functional dependencies* reflect the extent to which an individual can perform essential tasks to meet personal needs, such as eating, bathing, or toileting. At the time of an acute episode, function may be impaired due to some combination of new and old conditions such as developmental abnormalities, advanced cardiomyopathy, or an old stroke.

The impact of any illness or injury depends on both the acute episode and an individual's "foundation" at the time that the illness or injury arises. At the time of illness and injury, individuals may vary widely in their underlying foundations. Those affected by chronic diseases, aging, developmental or functional disturbances, and various psychosocial problems often have significantly disordered foundations. Those with impaired foundations are likely to take longer to recover functionally from their illness or injury, and may be more susceptible to the unfavorable impact of subsequent illness or injury.

The Essential "Triad"

Thus, subacute care represents care for different individuals who may have varying consequences of a relatively few common causes. The specific treatment or service (for example, wound or ventilator care) sufficiently defines neither the individual's needs nor the appropriate scope of the care.

Therefore, subacute care must also consider the same key elements known to influence outcomes: severity of illness, comorbidity, and functional dependency. There is evidence to suggest that patients may be best viewed by their various combinations of these factors (Rosenthal, Halloran, Kiley, et al., 1992). In other words, they may be grouped into a few basic "clusters," regardless of their underlying diagnoses or the site providing their care. For example, some ventilator patients need substantial Activities of Daily Living (ADL) support but not much medical or nursing care, while others have multiple medical complications with varying degrees of functional impairments. Other common examples of those with combinations of factors include:

- A stroke patient with a history of a heart condition, but with minimally impaired function from either condition
- A hip fracture patient with Parkinsonism and arthritis
- A COPD patient with diabetes and liver disease
- A pneumonia patient with delirium or dementia
- A patient with diverticulosis and other chronic conditions who recently had significant GI bleeding, who is no longer bleeding but is now debilitated
- A patient who suffered a massive stroke and is now dependent in most ADLs and is medically stable, but has other currently inactive problems, including heart disease and diabetes
- An end-stage heart-failure patient with recurrent bouts of pulmonary edema and limited activity tolerance

On the other hand, subacute programs also have been used to provide ongoing care for individuals who need some ongoing treatment, but do not necessarily have significant severity of illness, comorbidities, or dependencies. Examples of such patients include a young ambulatory individual who is still receiving antibiotics for osteomyelitis but who otherwise has few other health problems, or an uncomplicated cancer patient receiving chemotherapy.

DEFINING SUBACUTE CARE

While subacute care does not introduce any new care components into the health care system, it represents a definable approach to providing care to those who require a specific package of medical, nursing, and related services. Based on the preceding, subacute care may be viewed as care:

1) rendered immediately after, or instead of, acute hospitalization *(when given)*

2) to treat active medical conditions or to administer various treatments in the context of the patient's general condition, underlying foundation, and personal goals *(reason)*,

3) requiring the coordinated services of physicians, nurses, and other relevant professionals trained and knowledgeable in assessing and managing these conditions and administering the procedures *(by whom)*,

4) given as part of a specifically defined program regardless of the site *(site)*,

5) requiring frequent (daily to weekly) recurrent patient assessment and review of the clinical course and treatment plan *(frequency)*

6) combining aspects of the care of those with chronic illness or disability, functional impairment, and low or moderate acuity conditions *(intensity)*,

7) for a limited (several days to several months) time, or until a condition is stabilized or a predetermined treatment course is completed *(duration)*.

COMMON CLINICAL PROGRAMS

Subacute units may be general or specialized. For marketing purposes—and sometimes to organize the care—subacute care is often approached as a series of common conditions or syndromes with their own components and objectives (Table 2.5). Inevitably, there is some overlap among these services and patients. For example, patients in many service categories receive some rehabilitation therapies, and a pediatric service might provide elements of head injury care, postoperative care, and ventilator care. A predominant service need for one individual may be a secondary need for another. Thus, different programs treat comparable patients in programs or services of different names. Subacute care shares many of the features and patients of such programs as rehabilitation hospitals, transitional

TABLE 2.5 Common Subacute Care Programs

- AIDS care
- Cardiac recovery
- Dialysis/Renal failure
- Medically complex care: general/oncology-cancer care/pain management/hospice/terminal care
- Orthopedic care
- Pediatric care
- Post-operative care
- Psychiatric care
- Pulmonary care
- Rehabilitation services: general/brain and spinal cord injury/burns/stroke/trauma
- Wound care

Note: From *Subacute and Transitional Care Handbook* (p. 92), by S. A. Levenson, 1996. St. Louis: Beverly-Cracom.

care units, chronic or long-term hospitals, extended care facilities, and traditional Skilled Nursing Facilities (SNFs). The program's name or the designated bed or licensure level is thus less important than the characteristics and needs of the patients, and the availability of essential processes and services.

SUBACUTE CARE AS AN INTERDISCIPLINARY UNDERTAKING

The Participants

Subacute care's many players may be classified as providers and recipients. Providers may be categorized as owners and owner representatives (governing bodies or boards); management (chief executive officers [CEOs], administrators, and program directors); clinical leadership; practitioners; and support staff. Recipients include patients, families, and others who directly or indirectly support or influence either group (for example, payers).

Core practitioners and care providers in subacute care include activities or recreational therapists, clinical pharmacists, dietitians and nutritionists, generalist and specialist physicians, nurses, nursing assistants, social workers, and physical and occupational therapists. Other participants and practitioners may include clergy, dentists, ethicists, neuropsychologists, and respiratory and speech therapists. Health care support players include owners, boards of directors, chief executives and administrators, department heads, internal case managers, and support staff, such as housekeeping, maintenance, and dietary departments.

The "Team" Approach

Health care delivery is sometimes plagued by the lack of skilled individuals, and often damaged by the use of the wrong conceptual models to organize and manage care provision. Successful subacute care depends on organizing skilled individuals under the proper approach.

Like hospital care, subacute care requires more than one individual or discipline to meet diverse patient needs. It represents a package of services delivered systematically and repeatedly, within a limited time frame, by various individuals whose roles and activities must be coordinated appropriately. It reflects the successful performance of a series of care processes common to all health care settings (Table 2.6), which are needed to varying degrees. Its success also depends on effective support systems and management processes.

Thus, subacute care is best viewed as an interdisciplinary effort involving all parties, not just by those—such as nurses and physicians—who directly give the care. Subacute organization and operations should be influenced by the "total quality management" philosophy, which suggests that any enterprise's success in delivering high-quality products or services reflects the combined efforts of those who are directly or indirectly involved in, or who influence, a system (Rosenstein, 1996).

Subacute care combines aspects of acute medical, long-term nursing, and rehabilitative care (Table 2.7). Like much of the health care system, organizations and subacute care programs have their own identifiable culture (Kritchevsky & Simmons, 1991). Each program must establish an appropriate "culture," incorporating relevant aspects of these various approaches to care, and coordinating the input and performance of all the aforementioned participants. To date, only some programs have managed successfully to achieve this integration. Others have struggled to achieve the flexibility of managing patients with such varied combinations of needs and problems. In many programs, therapists, dietitians, nurses, and others accustomed to treating symptoms and managing problems based on the mandates of the Minimum Data Set (MDS) are having trouble understanding the critical concepts of treating causes before or while addressing consequences. There appears to be considerable room for improvement in the teaching and training of health care practitioners and managers about the attributes and performance required for a truly coordinated, integrated approach to care.

Individual practitioner and staff roles in caring for subacute patients may differ from roles in other situations, even though they may be practicing the same professions, giving the same treatments, and managing the same diseases. For example, since subacute patients have a recent or current acute illness, physicians must use their skills in diagnosis and treatment selection. However, a physician may need to aggressively manage an acute medical complication in one subacute patient, consult on another, and simply oversee a stable therapeutic regimen in a third. Secondary prevention—including the avoidance of iatrogenic and nosocomial complications—should always be a major consideration. The scope and aggressiveness of care should always be in the context of the patient's overall status, prognosis, and wishes. Rehabilitation and other therapies must be coordinated with the identification and treatment of the causes of functional impairments (Singleton, 1995).

TABLE 2.6 The Essential Processes of Subacute Care

Process	Objectives
Patient selection	• Decide whether individual needs subacute services • Determine whether the program can meet the patient's needs
Post-selection/preadmission	• Provide relevant and required information to the patient/family • Inform and prepare appropriate staff to accept the admission
Assessment	• Collect information about the individual that allows proper definition of their problems
Problem definition	• Correctly and completely define the individual's current status, including problems and deficits
Cause-and-effect analysis	• Correctly link the causes (disease states or other problems) of an individual's various problems to each other and to the problems themselves
Identifying care goals and objectives	• Correctly and completely define the purpose of giving care and the criteria that will be used to determine when the objectives have been met
Care planning	• Create a plan to address the individual's problems, including the responsibilities of various individuals and disciplines
Management of known problems	• Identify and implement appropriate treatment alternatives to address the individual's primary (main reason for admission) and secondary (coexisting) problems
Management of new problems/complications	• Identify and manage problems that arise as a result of existing conditions or that did not exist previously
Prevention of nosocomial/iatrogenic problems	• Identify areas of high risk and potential problems that may arise as a result of medications and treatments, or by being in a health care facility, and institute measures to try to prevent those problems and to recognize them if they arise despite precautions
Preparation for completion of treatment course	• Monitor responses to treatment and progress towards discharge • Plan for discharge and transfer by ensuring appropriate transfer site, follow up of problems, and communication of information to the patient and family, and others who will be providing continuing care
Follow-up	• Review care outcomes for the subacute stay and for a period of time after discharge • Review problems, concerns based on input of the providers and recipients of the care

Note: From *Subacute and Transitional Care Handbook* (p. 181), by S. A. Levenson, 1996. St. Louis: Beverly-Cracom.

TABLE 2.7 Features of Relevant "Cultures" That Must Be Blended in Subacute Care Programs

Care type	Features
Acute medical	• Quick, frequent, intensive interventions • Aggressively treatment-oriented • Rapid response to any condition changes • Frequent testing • Patients relatively uninvolved in decision making • Physician-intensive • Plentiful resources as needed • Multiple practitioners with relatively little coordination • Few mandatory care standards • Mostly short-stay patients
Long-term nursing	• Nursing- and nursing assistant-intensive • Primarily focused on ADL support and supervision • Less aggressive treatment and testing • Individuals and families more involved in decision making • Interdisciplinary team approach • Many mandatory performance and care standards • Both long- and short-stay patients • Relatively slow response to changing conditions
Rehabilitative	• Interdisciplinary team approach • Emphasis on managing consequences of illness and injury • Includes patients and families • Encourages patient participation and autonomy

Note: From *Subacute and Transitional Care Handbook*, by S. A. Levenson, 1996. St. Louis: Beverly-Cracom.

Practitioner Roles and Attributes

Effective subacute care requires practitioners who can perform various relevant functions (Table 2.8). They may do these things directly (by providing the care) or indirectly (by giving other practitioners appropriate support and guidance).

Many physicians appear to be uncertain about their appropriate role in the care of subacute patients. Some of them confuse subacute with long-term care, or are uncomfortable with a broader role beyond diagnosing and treating disease or performing procedures. Other, less familiar but equally valuable roles are to address new complications or condition

TABLE 2.8   Examples of the Various Roles of Subacute Practitioners

- Address both the causes and the consequences of illness and functional impairment
- Assess and treat acute and chronic illnesses
- Manage behavioral and functional impairments
- Help patients and families cope with the psychosocial or economic consequences of the current condition
- Manage a progressive decline possibly ending in death

changes; to clarify medical issues for patients, families and staff; to identify and manage complications or side effects of medications and treatments; to discuss the appropriate intensity and scope of medical care desired by a patient or family; to help justify a continued stay or the need for various tests or treatments; to clarify essential post-discharge services and support; to assess patient responses to treatment; and to identify and manage the causes of various patient problems. Like all participants, they must be flexible enough to alter their participation according to the demands of the situation and setting.

Attending physicians for subacute patients may be either primary care physicians or specialists. However, each may have certain strengths and weaknesses. Specialists (e.g., orthopedists, nephrologists, cardiologists) may have a more in-depth understanding of the technical aspects of performing procedures or of managing complicated problems related to a single organ system. Generalists may better understand the overall patient management, be better able to place the medical care in the context of the patient's overall treatment plan, appreciate the difference between treating an illness and solving a problem, and understand better how to help the staff, patients, and families deal with ethical and psychosocial issues.

Nurse practitioners (NPs) and physician assistants (PAs) also play a valuable role in providing subacute care. Nurse practitioners are nurses whose training also includes the medical model of diagnosis and treatment. Physician assistants are individuals who are trained to perform the typical functions of physicians, diagnosing and treating illness and performing technical procedures consistent with their skills. In subacute programs, the potential roles of NPs and PAs are largely interchangeable. They are usually either hired by the program or employed by individual physicians with patients on the unit.

NPs and PAs perform many routine and episodic assessments that require expertise between that of a nurse and a physician. They can assess acute condition changes, such as confusion or fever, and help a physician decide on the urgency and causes of an acute problem. They may also perform the initial history and physical, participate in interdisciplinary team conferences, review drug regimens, and educate patients, families, and staff.

PROVIDER REQUIREMENTS FOR SUBACUTE CARE

Subacute providers should be expected to provide effective, efficient care to all of their patients. The ability to deliver treatments or follow-up medical care for an acute illness is only one component of that care. Providers should be able to assess and manage individuals' physical, functional, and psychosocial needs.

So far, the licensure and regulation of subacute care have not evolved very far. Most subacute settings are regulated as Skilled Nursing Facilities under the federal OBRA '87 regulations, and licensed under state regulations regarding such facilities (Elon, 1995). While considering the various options, few states have identified the need to tailor regulations towards the level and scope of the care rather than the setting. It is unclear whether many state survey agencies yet understand the hybrid nature of subacute care and the importance of modifying traditional long-term care standards.

Subacute care is delivered in several distinct settings, including hospital-based and freestanding Skilled Nursing Facilities, long-term and chronic hospitals, and specialized rehabilitation facilities. Some aspects of acute or postacute care are also being given in the home and other noninstitutional settings.

All subacute settings do essentially the same things to different degrees or in different combinations for a few distinct populations of individuals. They offer a core of several dozen treatments, and they manage several dozen common primary medical conditions and many other occasional illnesses. They all must perform basic care processes such as assessment, problem definition, and treatment delivery. They tend to provide a limited number of treatments and procedures, few of them complex or of high risk (Table 2.9).

Ultimately, all subacute providers should be able to perform appropriate functions and achieve comparable outcomes for comparable patient populations. For example, they must perform the relevant care processes (assessment, problem identification, problem management, etc.); identify and manage *all* relevant dimensions of patient needs (physical, functional, and psychosocial); and not cause additional problems (for example, by failing to address relevant comorbidities, such as cardiac problems or skin breakdown in the rehabilitation patient). To expect less is to perpetuate a system where patients may receive disparate care for the same problem

TABLE 2.9 Common Treatments and Procedures in Subacute Patients

A. Medication administration
- Chemotherapy administration
- Intravenous medication administration
- IM/SQ medication administration

B. Administration of nutrients/fluids
- Hyperalimentation (TPN)
- Intravenous fluid administration
- Tube feeding

C. Non-medication treatments
- Blood transfusion
- Hemodialysis/Peritoneal dialysis
- Occupational therapy
- Physical therapy
- Respiratory, oxygen, medical gas therapy
- Specialty beds
- Speech/Language therapy
- Suctioning
- Ventilator care
- Ventilator weaning process
- Wound/Decubitus care (Stage III & IV)

D. Insertion of tubes/catheters to enable treatments
- Insertion of central IV
- Insertion of peripheral IV line

E. Care of tubes/catheters inserted to enable treatments and care
- Chest tube drainage
- Drainage tube (Other than chest tube or Foley catheter)
- Percutaneous catheters
- Tracheostomy care
- Management of peripheral or central IV lines

F. Monitoring
- Suicide precautions
- Blood gas monitoring
- Communicable disease care/Isolation

Note: From *Subacute and Transitional Care Handbook* (pp. 92–93), by S. A. Levenson, 1996. St. Louis: Beverly-Cracom.

depending on the site, the geographic location, and the bed licensure category.

Use of a more patient-oriented approach should make it possible to compare the outcomes of various patient clusters across different licensure categories and bed types. As acute care increasingly is provided outside of acute care hospitals, assessing the outcomes of various clusters across settings would help determine whether different providers and sites can provide comparable care and can also achieve similar outcomes for comparable patients. Their performance and their patient outcomes can then also be more readily compared. Providers may then differentiate themselves primarily on their efficiency and competence in accomplishing those outcomes. It should be possible to consolidate settings and licensure categories. For example, it may ultimately be unnecessary to designate separate medical and rehabilitation settings for the management of most patients.

REIMBURSEMENT FOR SUBACUTE CARE

There are currently several different categories of payers for subacute providers. Various payers appear to use significantly different methods for figuring appropriate reimbursement, resulting in significantly different payments for comparable care in different settings. The "average" cost approach probably does not accurately reflect the various clusters of patients comprising that average. A patient-based reimbursement methodology should help improve on some of the weaknesses of the current approach.

Currently, subacute care is reimbursed through several different provider types (primarily Medicare, Medicaid, private insurers, managed care) and in several different ways (primarily case-rate or per diem). The factors contributing to care costs at various sites can be identified (Table 2.10).

Several economic forces have driven the movement to subacute care. Because of the high cost of delivering services in hospitals, payers—especially managed care organizations—have sought less costly alternatives. As providers have had to share more of the financial risks of care, they have tried to lower their care delivery costs. These goals have encouraged increasing utilization of non-hospital settings to manage moderately complex problems without so much high-technology equipment and so many costly practitioners and support staff. Thus, subacute care also represents a merging of the goals of providers and payers.

TABLE 2.10 Factors Relating to Costs of Care

Direct care costs
- Skilled nursing personnel
- Nursing support staff
- Other clinical staff
- Technical support staff

Facility-related cost centers
- Plant operations, maintenance, repairs, etc.

General services costs
- Laundry, housekeeping, administration, etc.

Capital costs

Ancillaries
- *To treat functional impairments*
  Physical therapy/Occupational therapy/Speech therapy
- *To treat medical conditions*
  Medications
  IV therapies
  Oxygen/inhalation therapy
  Respiratory therapy
  Medical supplies
  Complex medical equipment
- *To monitor patients/define causes of problems*
  Radiology
  Laboratory
  Electrocardiography
  Complex medical equipment

Subacute care is also influenced by the trend towards managed care and the increasing emphasis on efficiency. However, like many others, managed care organizations are often still focusing on diagnoses and treatments, and may not appreciate the contribution of multiple factors to both outcomes and care costs. As discussed above, the primary diagnosis related to the acute episode or the primary treatment reason for authorizing subacute care may be influenced or overshadowed by other problems. Pertinent problems (depression, skin condition, nutritional status, etc.) that are not addressed in a timely fashion may result in persistent or recurrent problems that eventually cost even more to manage. Thus, payers should collaborate with practitioners to balance financial and quality considerations. The latter must be based upon correctly identifying and addressing the patient characteristics and provider processes that heavily influence outcomes. The same essential patient management principles should be incorporated throughout the care continuum, regardless of who pays for the care.

To date, many health care networks still do not achieve a true patient-oriented care continuum. Despite owning or affiliating with postacute and home care sites, there is still significant duplication and inadequate coordination of effort. True integration has also been stymied by reimbursement methodologies that are primarily diagnosis-, provider-, or treatment-based, not patient-based. Reimbursing different providers separately for care related to the same episode of illness has tended to encourage substantial duplication of effort.

The current health care delivery and reimbursement systems may inhibit market forces from playing more of a role in lowering costs. Reimbursement for treating the same condition or overall collection of problems may be radically different depending on the site, but not necessarily because of superior results. Care is reimbursed despite outcomes or minimal justification of same, and there are few consequences for inadequate or inappropriate care. The amount of reimbursement may be misaligned with the scope, intensity, or frequency of patient needs. The tendency to aggregate patient populations for reimbursement purposes, or to use an average payment for all patients in some settings, is likely to misrepresent the realities of the care, the costs of providing care, and the patient outcomes, unless a provider has a relatively homogeneous population.

Currently, there is a federal move to initiate in 1998, a prospective payment system (PPS) for skilled nursing care, possibly eventually linked to care at other sites for other phases of the same episode of illness. While not identifying a subacute payment category, the PPS will cover all subacute programs caring for Medicare patients. It is anticipated that a national prospective case-mix payment system would be more sensitive to the costs of meeting an individual's needs and equitable across all providers and settings. It would promote quality care, be based on costs, and be easy to administer. It would also ensure beneficiary access to appropriate services, help make those requiring more care to be desirable to facilities, and allow for quality measurements to be derived from the same instrument used to determine payment rates.

A valid patient-oriented approach would enable application of comparable measurements to other providers and settings. Preliminary data suggest that combinations of acuity, comorbidity, and dependency might be applicable in a prospective payment system to predict care costs (Jette et al., 1987). Such an approach would allow the same data elements to be used as a basis for both reimbursement and outcomes measurements across the care continuum, including home care and even acute hospital care.

PREDICTING FUTURE NEEDS FOR SUBACUTE SERVICES

Various developments will influence the bed need for subacute patients. These include the possible further development of technologies to improve monitoring and treatment capabilities of non-hospital sites such as homes and nursing facilities; greater physician willingness to practice in non-hospital settings; changes in reimbursement methodologies; and better integration of the management of the physical, social, functional, and ethical issues that impact subsequent placement and care choices.

Currently, subacute care sites provide care primarily after hospitalization, and SNF care is not covered under Medicare without a qualifying hospital stay. However, not being subject to the 3-day stay rule, managed care payers are increasingly bypassing hospitals for direct subacute admissions. Therefore, another significant development will be progressive shifts in reimbursement methodologies that allow subacute sites to care directly for certain acute medical conditions instead of first requiring hospitalization. Many individuals with progressive physical condition changes or relatively uncomplicated acute illnesses—especially the frail elderly—could receive necessary diagnostics and treatment without being hospitalized.

A possible obstacle to the expanded use of subacute settings is the continuation of site-specific regulations that fail to recognize the various levels of care within the same setting, or that unnecessarily limit the provision of comparable care in different settings. This could be remedied by modifying regulations to primarily address levels of care before considering the care site.

SUMMARY

In many ways, subacute care represents a model for the changing U.S. health care environment, illustrating important principles regarding medical illness, health care service delivery, regulations, physician practice, and reimbursement. It shows that service delivery is often no longer strictly associated with a discrete care site and that all providers—regardless of site—perform common functions and need common standards to manage patients of comparable status. It confirms that medical illness has various aspects and influences, and that medical management alone is often insufficient to produce a desired outcome when the acute condition has a broad impact or the individual's "foundation" is compromised. It reinforces the need for a patient-oriented, problem-oriented approach to both the delivery and reimbursement of care. It reflects how strongly reimbursement impacts the scope and adequacy of care, and how reimbursement methodologies may need to be based on a new model reflecting patient needs more than sites or practitioners. Hopefully, these issues will receive the serious attention they deserve from practitioners, providers, academicians, government officials, and payers.

REFERENCES

Bernardini, B., Meinecke, C., Pagani, M., Grillo, A., Fabbrini, S., Zaccarini, C., Corsini, C., Scapellato, F., & Bonaccorso, O. (1995). Comorbidity and adverse clinical events in the rehabilitation of older adults after hip fracture. *Journal of the American Geriatrics Society, 43*, 894–898.

Ceder, L., Thorngren, K. G., & Wallden, B. (1980). Prognostic indicators and early home rehabilitation in elderly patients with hip fracture. *Clinical Orthopedics, 152*, 173–184.

Cleves, M. A., Sanchez, N., & Draheim, M. (1997). Evaluation of two competing methods for calculating Charlson's comorbidity index when analyzing short-term mortality using administrative data. *Journal of Clinical Epidemiology, 50*, 903–908.

Elon, R. D. (1995). Medical practice in nursing facilities: Assessing the Impact of OBRA. In P. R. Katz, R. L. Kane, and M. S. Mezey (Eds.), *Quality care in geriatric settings*. New York: Springer Publishing Co.

Greenfield, S., Apolone, G., McNeil, B. J., & Cleary, P. D. (1993). The importance of co-existent disease in the occurrence of postoperative complications and one-year recovery in patients undergoing total hip replacement: Comorbidity and outcomes after hip replacement. *Medical Care, 31*, 141–154.

Hoenig, H., Nusbaum, N., & Brummel-Smith, K. (1997). Geriatric rehabilitation: State of the Art. *Journal of the American Geriatric Society, 45*, 1371–1381.

Incalzi, A. R., Capparella, O., Gemma, A., Porcedda, P., Raccis, G., Jommella, L., & Carbonin, P. U. (1992). A simple method of recognizing geriatric patients at risk for death and disability. *Journal of the American Geriatric Society, 40*, 34–38.

Jette, S. M., Harris, B. A., Clearly, P. D., & Campion, E. W. (1987). Functional recovery after hip fracture. *Archives of Physical Medicine and Rehabilitation, 68*, 735–740.

Kritchevsky, S. B., & Simmons, B. P. (1991). Continuous quality improvement: Concepts and applications for physician care. *JAMA, 266*, 1817–1823.

Levenson, S. A. (1996). *Subacute and transitional care handbook*. St. Louis: Beverly-Cracom.

Liu, M., Domen, K., & Chino, N. (1997). Comorbidity measures for stroke outcome research: A preliminary study. *Archives of Physical Medicine and Rehabilitation, 78*, 166–172.

Magaziner, J., Simonick, E. M., Kashner, T. M., Hebel, J. R., & Kenzora, J. E. (1990). Predictors of functional recovery one year following hospital discharge for hip fracture: A prospective study. *Journal of Gerontology, 45*, 101–107.

Moos, R. H., & Mertens, J. R. (1996). Patterns of diagnoses, comorbidities, and treatment in late-middle-aged and older affective disorder patients: Comparison of mental health and medical sectors. *Journal of the American Geriatric Society, 44*, 682–688.

Muder, R. R., Brennen, C., Swenson, D. L., & Wagener, M. (1996). Pneumonia in a long-term care facility: A prospective study of outcome. *Archives of Internal Medicine, 156*, 2365–2370.

Newschaffer, C. J., Bush, T. L., & Penberthy, L. T. (1997). Comorbidity measurement in elderly female breast cancer patients with administrative and medical records data. *Journal of Clinical Epidemiology, 50*, 725–733.

O'Keeffe, S., & Lavan, J. (1997). The prognostic significance of delirium in older hospital patients. *Journal of the American Geriatric Society, 45*, 174–178.

Parmelee, P. A., Thuras, P. D., Katz, I. R., & Lawton, M. P. (1995). Validation of the cumulative illness rating scale in a geriatric residential population. *Journal of the American Geriatric Society, 43*, 130-137.

Poses, R. M., McClish, D. K., Smith, W. R., Bekes, C., & Scott, W. E. (1996). Prediction of survival of critically ill patients by admission comorbidity. *Journal of Clinical Epidemiology, 49*, 743–747.

Presented to the American Health Care Association, 10/96.

Rochon, P. A., Katz, J. N., Morrow, L. A., McGlinchey-Berroth, R., Ahlquist, M. M., Sarkarati, M., & Minaker, K. L. (1996). Comorbid illness is associated with survival and length of hospital stay in patients with chronic disability: A prospective comparison of three comorbidity indices. *Medical Care, 34*, 1093–1101.

Rosenstein, R. (1996). *Subacute care project: Progress report*. Baltimore, MD: Maryland Health Resources Planning Commission.

Rosenthal, G. E., Halloran, E. J., Kiley, M., & Landefeld, C. S. (1995). Predictive validity of the nursing severity index in patients with musculoskeletal disease. *Journal of Clinical Epidemiology, 48*, 179–188.

Rosenthal, G. E., Halloran, E. J., Kiley, M., Pinkley, C., & Landefeld, C. S. (1992). Development and validation of the Nursing Severity Index. A new method for measuring severity of illness using nursing diagnoses. *Medical Care, 30*, 1127–1141.

Satish, S., Winograd, C. H., Chavez, C., & Bloch, D. A. (1996). Geriatric targeting criteria as predictors of survival and health care utilization. *Journal of the American Geriatric Society, 44*, 914–921.

Singleton, G. (1995). Overcoming culture conflict. *Provider, 21*, 27–30.

Zureik, M., Lombrail, P., Davido, A., Trouillet, J. L., Tran, B., Levy, A., & Lang, T. (1997). Predicting the outcome in elderly patients of hospital admission for acute care in Paris, France: construction and initial validation of a simple index. *Journal of Epidemiology and Community Health, 51*, 192–198.

3
From Post-Acute to Chronic Care: Cost and Policy Implications of Medicare Home Health Expansion

Penny Hollander Feldman

Home health services—ranging from skilled nursing and physical therapy to hands-on personal care—have grown dramatically over the last decade. Originally a token Medicare benefit intended to keep hospital costs from "going through the roof" (Benjamin, 1993), by 1996 home care accounted for more than $18 billion, or 9% of the Medicare budget (Prospective Payment Commission [ProPAC], 1997). Moreover, the Medicare program has become the largest source of payment for home-based services (Vladeck & Miller, 1994). As a result, home health spending has risen to the top of the Medicare policy agenda, eliciting difficult questions about the appropriateness and efficacy of services and the likely effects of emerging cost-containment proposals.

This chapter reviews what is known about the growth of Medicare home health expenditures in recent years. In particular, it focuses on the expansion of the Medicare home health benefit from post-acute to chronic care and on the policy implications of that expansion. The chapter addresses four main questions:

1) How has the Medicare home health benefit evolved;

2) What are the components and causes of Medicare home health expenditure growth;
3) How has available research on home health outcomes and variations influenced the terms of the policy debate; and
4) What is the potential for improving home health efficiency and constraining home health costs, while meeting the needs of Medicare beneficiaries.

EVOLUTION OF THE MEDICARE HOME HEALTH BENEFIT

Despite efforts of the Health Care Financing Administration (HCFA) to clarify key statutory provisions, the Medicare home health benefit is complex, vague, and subject to multiple interpretations (Vladeck & Miller, 1994). For a period of roughly two decades it was essentially restricted to short-term post-acute care primarily through skilled nursing or therapy services (Benjamin, 1993). Supportive or so-called "unskilled" services (i.e., personal care provided by a home health aide) were incidental to skilled services, and could be provided only in conjunction with them. Today, although skilled short-term care is still the dominant paradigm for describing the Medicare home health model, the reality has changed. Since 1988, when HCFA settled a class action suit brought by a coalition of Medicare home health users, providers, and members of Congress (Duggan v Bowen, 1988), the statutory language has been interpreted more permissively to allow the provision of care on a long-term basis to individuals who qualify under an expanded definition of skilled nursing needs. Moreover, the care provided can and often does include a substantial amount of home health aide services.

Medicare home health is covered under both Part A (hospital insurance benefits) and Part B (supplementary medical insurance benefits).[1] To be eligible under either part, a beneficiary must be homebound, under the care of a physician, and in need of *skilled* care—defined as physical therapy, speech therapy, intermittent skilled nursing services, or continuous occupational therapy. Once these conditions have been met, an individual may also receive medical social services, durable medical equipment

---

[1]In recent years, most home health services have been financed through Part A, with Part B covering home health only for beneficiaries who did not have Part A. However, as a result of the Balanced Budget Act of 1997 (PL105-33) starting in January 1998, Part A will cover only post-institutional home health services for up to 100 visits. All remaining home health visits (those not following a 3-day institutional stay and all post-institutional visits after the first 100) will be covered by Part B.

(subject to a 20% copayment), and home health aide services. So long as they are medically "reasonable and necessary" for treatment of an illness or injury and certified by a physician every 60 days, none of these services are limited to a specific time period (e.g., post-hospital) or to a visit ceiling (Vladeck & Miller, 1994).

Medicare home health benefits were not always so generous. Until Congress enacted the Social Security Amendments of 1972 (P.L. 92-603), there was a 20% copayment for home health services covered under Part B. Furthermore, until enactment of the Omnibus Reconciliation Act (ORA) of 1980 (P.L. 96-499), visits were limited to 100 under both Parts A and B; Part A required a 3-day prior hospital stay; and Part B required that beneficiaries satisfy the Part B deductible before home health payments could be initiated (Silverman, 1990). ORA removed these restrictions and expanded opportunities for for-profit agencies to become Medicare-certified. These legislative changes were associated with rapid service growth during the period 1974 to 1984 (Silverman, 1990). During that period, the proportion of beneficiaries receiving home health services tripled, from 16 to 50 per 1000 enrollees, while the actual number of home health users climbed from about 393 thousand to 1.5 million. Concomitantly, Medicare home health payments increased from about $141 million in 1974 to $1.9 billion in 1984 (Helbing, Sangl, & Silverman, 1992).

Despite, or perhaps because of, a decade of expansion, home health growth suddenly ceased in the mid-1980s. Responding to investigations by the General Accounting Office and by HCFA suggesting that as many as 30% of home health claims approved for payment might be inappropriate, Medicare's intermediaries intensified their review and greatly increased their retrospective denial of home health claims in 1986 and 1987 (Bishop & Skwara, 1993; Helbing et al., 1992; Silverman, 1990). By 1987, the total number of Medicare home health users had stabilized at about 1.5 million, the number of visits per person served had dropped from 28 (in 1983) to 23, and home health payments had stabilized at about $1.9 billion (Table 3.1).

Industry and consumer advocacy groups protested the sudden crackdown on claims and filed Duggan v Bowen, claiming 1) that HCFA was using an unlawfully restrictive definition of "part time or intermittent care" to deny benefits to qualified patients, and 2) that intermediaries operating without adequate supervision or regulations from HCFA were arbitrarily denying claims (Helbing et al., 1992). The court found for the plaintiffs, ruling that intermediaries in practice had been substituting "part-time *and* intermittent" for the statute's "part-time *or* intermittent" language and ordered HCFA to allow part-time care for as many as 7 days a week.

TABLE 3.1 Medicare Home Health Payments & Utilization 1983–1996

Year	Total Payments ($ Billion)	Total Payments Percent Change	Persons Served Persons Served (000)	Persons Served Percent Change	Visits per Person Served Visits/ User	Visits per Person Served Percent Change	Payment per Visit Payment per Visit ($)	Payment per Visit Percent Change
1983	1.6		1,318		28		43	
1984	1.9	18.8	1,498	13.7	27	−3.6	46	7.0
1985	1.9	0	1,549	3.4	25	−7.4	49	6.5
1986	1.9	0	1,571	1.4	24	−4.0	51	4.1
1987	1.9	0	1,544	−1.7	23	−4.2	54	5.9
1988	2.1	10.5	1,582	2.5	23	0	56	3.7
1989	2.6	23.8	1,685	6.5	27	17.4	56	0
1990	3.9	50.0	1,940	15.1	36	33.3	57	1.8
1991	5.6	46.0	2,223	14.6	45	25.0	56	−1.8
1992	7.9	38.6	2,523	13.5	54	20.0	58	3.6
1993	10.4	30.6	2,868	13.7	59	9.3	61	5.2
1994	13.5	30.2	3,175	10.7	70	18.6	61	—
1995	16.4	21.8	3,570	12.4	75	7.1	62	1.6
1996*	18.3	11.3	3,735	4.6	77	2.7	64	3.2

Source: ProPAC, June 1997, Tables 4-7 and C-4. Pages 111, 137.
*All 1996 figures are estimates.

As a result of this litigation, HCFA revised the eligibility and coverage sections of the home health agency manual (HIM-11). In addition to liberalizing the interpretation of "part-time or intermittent," it expanded the home health benefit in other important ways. The clarifications to the manual stated that intermediaries could not deny coverage based solely on utilization review screens and that physicians' orders for care had to be accepted unless contradicted by "objective clinical evidence." Coverage could not be denied solely on the grounds that a patient had a chronic disease or required long-term care, so long as skilled nursing care was required[2] (Helbing et al., 1992). Moreover, the definition of "skilled" was enlarged beyond the hands-on procedures (e.g., wound care, tube feeding) that had traditionally comprised skilled nursing care to include certain services requiring skilled nursing judgment. Under the revised HIM-

---

[2]Prior to the court's ruling, intermediaries sometimes used blanket rules to determine medical necessity. Also, some intermediaries denied coverage to an individual needing skilled care if the person's condition was stable and did not require intervention to foster rehabilitation or address a medical crisis.

11, individuals whose only nursing care need is for "skilled nursing observation" or for management of essential unskilled services provided by a paid or unpaid caregiver can now qualify for Medicare home health coverage and for the full range of services (including home health aide services) associated with home health eligibility. The practical import of these changes has been that the Medicare home health benefit is no longer confined to a relatively short course of care for recovery from an acute illness, but is available to beneficiaries with chronic conditions and ongoing skilled care needs (Bishop & Skwara, 1993; Cohen & Tumlinson, 1997). This expansion from post-acute to chronic care prepared the way for a period of rapid expenditure growth in the post-1988 period.

COMPONENTS AND CAUSES OF HOME HEALTH EXPENDITURE GROWTH

Home health expenditures have been the fastest growing item in the Medicare budget since the late 1980s. They rose from $1.9 billion in 1986 to an estimated $18.3 billion in 1996, an average annual growth rate of 25% (ProPAC, 1997). While home health was only 2.5% of the total Medicare program budget in 1986, it was estimated to be 9.1% in 1996, overtaking outpatient payments as a share of Medicare spending (Table 3.2).

What has been driving home health costs? The short answer to this question is that increased service use has been the driver. Between 1986 and 1996, the number of Medicare home health visits grew from 38

**TABLE 3.2 Expenditure Growth 1986–1996
Medicare Home Health, SNF & Outpatient Payments**

	$Billions		% Total Medicare $	
	1986	1996*	1986	1996*
Home Health	$ 1.9	$ 18.3	2.5	9.1
SNF	$ .6	$ 11.7	.79	5.8
Outpatient	$ 5.2	$ 16.6	6.7	8.3
Total Medicare	$75.7	$200.6	100%	

Source: Percentages computed from Prospective Payment Commission, Report to Congress, June 1997. Tables C-2 and C-4. Pages 136, 137.
*1996 figures are all estimates.

million to an estimated 286 million, a 750% increase (ProPAC, 1997).[3] Service use itself is a product of individual users and visits per user. The principal component responsible for recent expenditure growth has been a dramatic increase in the number of home health visits per user, from an average of 24 in 1986 to an average of 77 in 1996 (Table 3.1 and Figure 3.1). As can be seen from Figure 3.2, more than half (52%) of the average annual growth in home health payments since 1986 can be accounted for by an increase in the number of visits per person served. Nearly 40% of the increase is attributable to more beneficiaries receiving care, and only about 10% to an increase in Medicare payments per home health visit.[4,5] Increased service use reflects increases in both skilled and unskilled visits. However, unskilled service use has been rising more quickly. For example, between 1988 and 1993, average nursing visits per user roughly doubled, from 12 to 27, while average home health aide visits per user tripled, from 8 to 24 (Bishop, Skwara, & Sangl, 1995).

What are the underlying forces that have been fueling increased service use? A multitude of related and mutually reinforcing factors have been cited in the literature. First is expanding service capacity. The home health industry has low barriers to entry: little capital is needed for start-up, and certificate of need regulations have generally been less stringent than for investments in hospitals or nursing homes. Between 1990 and 1995 alone, there was a 50% increase in the number of Medicare-certified home health agencies, from 5793 to 8662 (ProPAC, 1996). Growth was fastest among for-profit agencies and next fastest among hospital-based agencies. A strong positive relationship between Medicare home health use and the number of home health agencies in an area has been well established in the literature, as has a similar relationship between home health use and the proportion of agencies that are for-profit (Benjamin, 1986; Cohen & Tumlinson, 1997; Kenney & Dubay, 1992; Schore, 1994; Swan & Benjamin, 1992).

Sustained pressure to reduce and even avert hospital stays generally is considered to be a second factor contributing to home health growth.

---

[3]In contrast, Medicare home health payment per visit grew 25.5%, and the number of persons served grew 237.8% (ProPac, 1997).

[4]This is unlike the period 1974–1988, when expenditure increases were attributable principally to increases in the number of Medicare enrollees, the proportion of enrollees served, and per visit costs. Between 1974 and 1983, visits per person served accounted for only 10.5% of the total increase in program payments, while between 1983 and 1988, they accounted for 31.8% (Silverman, 1990).

[5]The low growth rate in payments per visit may be somewhat misleading. This is because the composition of home health visits has changed over time such that unskilled home health aide visits now constitute a higher proportion of total visits than they did previously. Thus even though the cost per visit (for *all* types) has not risen significantly, Medicare is in essence purchasing a different product.

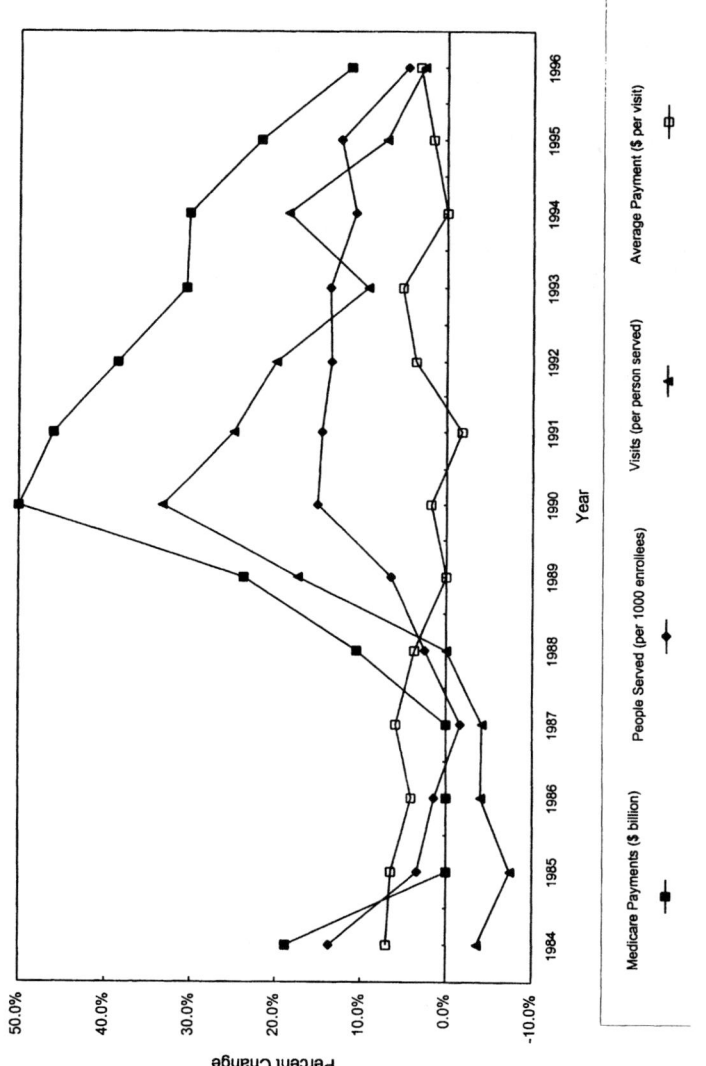

FIGURE 3.1 Medicare home health annual growth rates.

Source: PROPAC June 1997 Report to Congress.

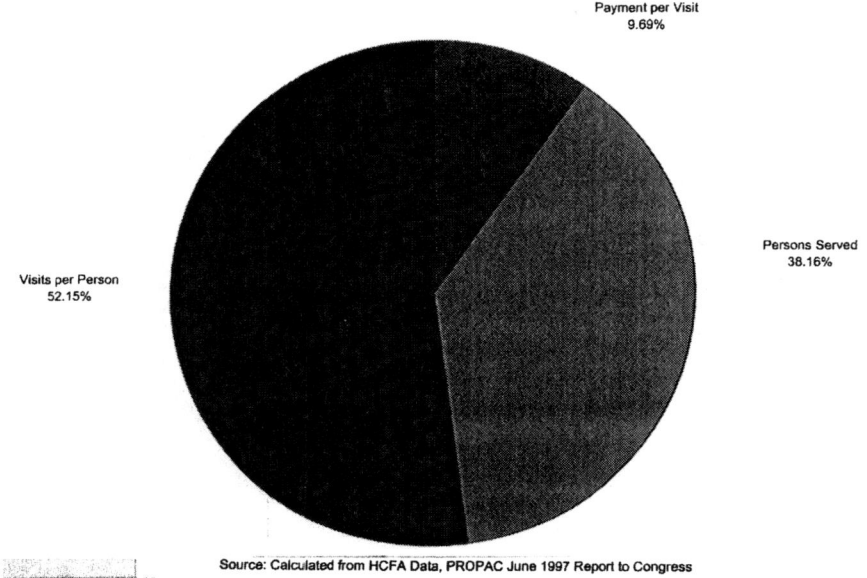

FIGURE 3.2 Components of growth in Medicare home health care 1986–1996 (average annual growth in total payments).

Hospital inpatient days fell on average 2.2% per year between 1988 and 1995. In the words of the Prospective Payment Commission, "The need and demand for post-acute care have grown as inpatient stays have been shortened and, for some beneficiaries, eliminated altogether" (ProPAC, 1996, p. 92).

A third and related contributing factor is the technological advances allowing home care for more complex conditions. Improvements in the safety of home infusion and intravenous therapy, for example, now permit a significant amount of high-tech care to be administered to patients with cancer, AIDS, end-stage congestive heart failure, and the like, outside of hospitals and physician offices (Congressional Research Service [CRS], 1996; Hastings Center, 1994; Mehlman & Youngner, 1991).

Cost-based payment is a fourth and powerful factor fueling home health use. Medicare payment methods have effectively restrained per-visit costs by subjecting them to an aggregate cost limit (Bishop & Skwara, 1993;

Silverman, 1990). Perhaps the simplest way for a home health agency to reduce per-visit costs is to spread fixed costs over a larger volume of services. Increasing volume, in turn, can be readily accomplished by providing more visits to needy patients who are already on the caseload, while at the same time obtaining more referrals. Thus the visit-based unit of payment has driven up total costs by rewarding agencies for providing more services (ProPAC, 1996).

A fifth, and some believe the major, factor underlying escalating service use are changes in the definition of the Medicare home health benefit made in response to Duggan *v* Bowen. With changes in coverage that allow longer episodes of care for people who continue to have skilled care needs, the Medicare home health benefit has come to straddle both the acute and long-term care service domains. Although most users of Medicare home health services receive care for a period of less than 120 days, a significant minority (approximately 25%) receive services for a much longer period of time—264 days on average, or nearly nine months (Goldberg & Schmitz, 1994). In 1994, 19% of Medicare home health users had 100 or more visits (HCFA Bureau of Data Management & Strategy, 1995), and 14% had more than 150 (Mauser, 1996). Although no precise data are available on the share of Medicare home health dollars going to chronically disabled enrollees, those with 100 or more visits accounted for approximately 63% of the total $13.6 billion that Medicare spent on home health in 1994 (HCFA Bureau of Data Management & Strategy, 1995). Thus, slightly less than a fifth of home health users accounted for over four-fifths of Medicare home health payments.

Finally, because the distribution of Medicare home health visits is shifting away from short-stay, low-visit users to long-stay, high-visit users with heavy reliance on home health aide services (Bishop & Skwara, 1993; Mauser, 1996) and because Medicaid traditionally has been viewed as the source of coverage for long-term care, policy makers and analysts are beginning to suspect that Medicare may be substituting for or overlapping with Medicaid-funded home care. Several studies have found a weak inverse relationship between per capita Medicare and Medicaid home health spending at the state level (Kane, Kane, Ladd, & Nielsen, 1995; Kenney, Coughlin, & Rimes, 1995; Miller, Mauser, & Harrington, 1995). Furthermore, in the most detailed study to date, Cohen and Tumlinson (1997) found that over a 3-year period (1991-93) both the number of Medicare home health users and the number of Medicare home health visits per user were significantly greater in states that faced greater fiscal pressure with respect to their Medicaid budgets (measured by Medicaid as a percentage of the state's budget), spent less on Medicaid home health programs, and lacked Medicaid personal care programs. They also found evidence that as the number of state long-term care (Intermediate Care Facility) beds decreased, the number of Medicare home health users increased, suggesting that the Medicare benefit was in fact serving individuals who might otherwise need to be institutionalized in an ICF.

Additional evidence suggests that long-stay, high-use Medicare home health patients have underlying functional impairments and ongoing supportive service needs associated with the chronic medical problems and acute exacerbations that render them eligible for Medicare home health services (Manton, Stallard, & Woodbury, 1994). Data from the 1992 Medicare Beneficiary Survey indicate that high-visit enrollees (those with 150 or more total visits) had on average more than twice as many limitations in activities of daily living as low-visit enrollees (2.64 versus 1.19 ADL limitations) and used thirteen times more aide visits (157 versus 12) (Mauser, 1996). High-visit enrollees were also more likely to be Medicaid eligible (40% of those with more than 150 visits in 1992, compared to only 22% of those with fewer than 150 visits) (Mauser & Miller, 1995). Thus while the relationship between Medicare and Medicaid-covered home health services is undoubtedly complex, it seems quite likely that policies determining eligibility and coverage for Medicare home health both influence and are influenced by Medicaid long-term care policy.

HOME CARE RESEARCH AND THE POLICY DEBATE

Although unusually rapid expenditure growth is almost invariably a target for the scrutiny of policy makers and politicians, accelerating growth per se is not necessarily undesirable, particularly if it reflects conscious policy choices or explicit decisions to elevate one set of priorities over another. Indeed, when Congress enacted the ORA provisions of 1980, the explicit intent was to increase home health service use. In 1982, a report of the Senate Committee on Labor and Human Resources expressed the view that

> Increased utilization of home health care should result in long-term federal cost savings through decreased nursing home and hospital admissions and shorter lengths of stay, as well as by increasing family support for the elderly. *Of equal importance* is the knowledge that increased availability of home health care will enable many elderly and *chronically ill persons* to maintain their independence and community ties and to lead lives of greater personal dignity and satisfaction [emphasis added] (quoted in Silverman, 1990, p. 116).

Additionally, the impending implementation of the Medicare hospital prospective payment system created the clear expectation that home health use would accelerate as hospitals faced incentives for earlier patient discharge.

If Medicare home health services were to be encouraged as a vehicle for both decreasing institutionalization and improving the quality of life of chronically ill persons, why then should the rapid utilization increases occurring between 1974 and 1984, and more recently, since 1988, have engendered such an outpouring of concern, not only among high-level officials and budget "watchdogs" but increasingly among analysts and researchers? Part of the answer to this question lies in the fact that improving quality of life for chronically ill persons has rarely received equal billing in the policy debate over Medicare home health. Contrary to the language of the Senate report quoted above, and more typical of observations about the Medicare home health benefit, is the language of a recent Congressional Research Service (CRS) Report prepared by the CRS's Education and Public Welfare Division. This report declares that

> Medicare's home health benefit is intended to serve beneficiaries needing acute *medical* care . . . and was never envisioned as providing coverage for the nonmedical supportive care and personal care assistance needed by chronically impaired persons (CRS, 1996, p. 1).

A major consequence of justifying home health care with rhetorical claims that it would produce cost savings on the institutional side is that the sorting out of claims about its impact has been a key feature of ongoing policy debate (Benjamin, 1993). Moreover, the dependence on institutional cost savings as a rationale for the benefit has served to undermine its legitimacy. This is because most of the home care research conducted over the last 15 years has focused on whether or not home-based services substitute for nursing home use, and has concluded that they do not. As early as 1980, Weissert, Wan, Livierqators, and Pellegrino (1980) reviewed the cost-effectiveness of homemaker services for the chronically ill and found evidence of increased rather than decreased costs. In the early 1980s, Congress funded the National Long-Term Care or Channeling Demonstration to evaluate community-based approaches as an alternative to institutional care, and by 1988 the findings of this study—that home care did not prevent nursing home use—were widely available (Kemper, 1988; Weissert, 1991). Between 1985 and 1995, a series of articles appearing in highly respected journals reviewed the field of home care research and uniformly reported mixed to negligible evidence supporting claims for home care as a cost-saving alternative to nursing home or hospital care (Benjamin, 1993; Hedrick & Inui, 1986; Hughes, 1985; Kane & Kane, 1987; Weissert & Hedrick, 1994; Weissert, Cready, & Pawelak, 1988).

Many of the studies included in these reviews focused on long-term, supportive services rather than on home *health* services per se, and the authors of the reviews rarely make the distinction. Several well-controlled studies of home health services recently have shown significant functional improvements and/or institutional cost savings for individuals within 60 days of home health admission (Shaughnessy, Schlenker, & Hittle, 1994); for severely disabled veterans (Hughes et al., 1990); for groups with chronic illnesses, such as congestive heart failure, who are at high risk of hospitalization (Rich et al., 1995); and for individuals receiving comprehensive geriatric assessment (Stuck et al., 1995). Furthermore, a recent meta-analysis focusing solely on the impact of home health care, narrowly defined, on hospital use, did find that home care had a small to moderate effect across a majority of studies—reducing hospital use from 2.5 to 6 days (Hughes et al., 1997). It is possible that as both research and critical reviews of the research literature become more sophisticated, focusing on illness trajectories and functional outcomes for well-delineated subgroups of patients and carefully specified interventions, the weight of evidence will shift in the direction of demonstrating the cost-effectiveness of home-based services. Such studies, however, will likely find that care is cost-effective in some instances and not in others, and will therefore imply the need for complex algorithms to identify those patients most likely to benefit from specific kinds of interventions (Kane, Finch, Blewett, Burns, & Moskowitz, 1994). Thus the conclusion seems inescapable that neither currently available nor future research will be able to support broad population-wide expansion of home health care solely or primarily on grounds of institutional cost savings.

Concerns about the purpose and cost-effectiveness of the Medicare home health benefit have been exacerbated, moreover, by emerging analyses of variations in home health use and expenditures across regions, states, and provider types. Long (1994) found significant regional variations in Medicare home health use after controlling for patient, area, and agency characteristics. Both numbers of visits and home health episode lengths were higher in the East South Central and West South Central regions than in other regions of the U.S. Yet regions with lower levels of use did not appear to have poorer patient outcomes, as measured by death, hospitalization, or readmission to home health.

HCFA (HCFR Medicare and Medicaid Statistical Supplement, 1995), the Office of the Inspector General (1995), the U.S. General Accounting Office (1996) and the Prospective Payment Commission (ProPAC, 1996) have all published recent studies of interstate variation. They have found roughly a five-fold difference in the range of persons served per 1000 enrollees, nearly a fifteen-fold difference in visits per enrollee, and a ninefold difference in average home health payments per enrollee (HCFR, 1995). Agencies with high visits per user were concentrated in five southern states: Alabama, Georgia, Louisiana, Mississippi, and Tennessee. Over 80% of home health agencies in these states exceeded the national average of 50 home health visits per beneficiary (Office of the Inspector General, 1995).

Four major factors have been cited as contributing causes to such dramatic interstate variation. First are differences in the number of agencies and, in particular, the proportion of for-profit agencies providing care in a given area. In virtually every study of agency type, for-profit agencies have been found to provide significantly more visits per user and per episode than non-profits or hospital-based agencies (Benjamin, 1986; Cohen & Tumlinson, 1997; Kenney & Dubay, 1992; ProPAC, 1996; Schore, 1994; Swan & Benjamin, 1992; Williams, 1994). Moreover, these differences hold up after controlling for the health and functional status of users, as well as age, sex, and living situation (Mauser, 1995). Because proprietary agencies provide a much higher proportion of care in the high-use South Central and South Atlantic states (Schore, 1994), their practice style has frequently been cited as a contributing cause of variation (Welch, Wennberg, & Welch, 1996).

Second is nursing home supply. Studies by Kenney and Dubay (1992) and Cohen and Tumlinson (1997) both found evidence that Medicare home health use is greater in states with fewer nursing home beds. The latter found that an increase of one skilled nursing facility in a state was associated with a decrease of 34 to 52 home health users per enrollee across a 3-year study period. They also found an inverse relationship between the number of long-term care (ICF) beds and the number of Medicare home health users.

A third contributing factor is thought to be state Medicaid policy. Of the five southern states with the highest Medicare home health visit rates, all fell below the 50th percentile nationally in Medicaid home and community-based care expenditures, and two (Tennessee and Mississippi) were at the very bottom. As noted above, at least one recent study has found evidence of an interaction between state Medicaid policies and Medicare home health use, where states with a high Medicaid burden or low Medicaid home care spending demonstrate higher numbers of Medicare home health users and visits (Cohen & Tumlinson, 1997).

A final contributing factor—related in part to states' long-term care supply and Medicaid polices—may be the underlying health of the population receiving Medicare home health services. Although most of the variation studies have not been able to use sophisticated controls for patients' health and functional status (because they relied on aggregate data), Schore (1994) found a higher incidence of chronic conditions such as diabetes, hypertension, and other cerebrovascular diseases among patients in the high-use South Central states. She concluded that "The South Central states may be using home health services as a type of long-term care, with above-average use of home health aide services and below-average use of therapy" (pp. 30–31).

In addition to the major factors discussed above, variation studies have attempted to control for a number of other variables posited to contribute to widespread differences in Medicare home health service use. These include area characteristics (e.g., urban/rural status, size of metropolitan area, and proportion of people living in poverty); health care/supply side variables (e.g., hospital occupancy rates, hospital beds per 1000 persons 65+, average length of hospital stay for people 65+, and percent hospitals with home health programs); state policy and program variables (e.g., state home care eligibility criteria, Medicaid home care reimbursement methodology, and number of home and community-based care waiver programs); and other population/patient characteristics (e.g., demographics, principal diagnosis, comorbid conditions, and prior service use). Even the best controlled studies, however, have explained barely half the variance in patterns of Medicare home health use (Cohen & Tumlinson, 1997). Thus significant unexplained variations remain, underscoring the lack of national consensus on the appropriate use of home health care (Welch et al., 1996) and contributing to the growing concern over escalating Medicare home health expenditures.

FUTURE POLICY DIRECTIONS

Medicare home health is at a critical juncture. The vast majority of home health users and episodes still fall into the category of post-acute care. However, the bulk of Medicare home health visits and the major growth in Medicare home health spending are attributable to the program's transition from a relatively restrictive post-acute benefit to a more expansive benefit providing substantial amounts of long-term care, much of it in the form of supportive services to persons with chronic illness. With the impending depletion of the Medicare Part A Trust Fund, which pays for almost all home health claims, pressure to constrain visits and costs is mounting. Voices in both legislative and executive bodies, in policy shops and in prominent journals are beginning to question whether Medicare is "institutionaliz[ing] societal 'caring' " and medicalizing services that may be only tangentially related to medical care (Welch et al., 1996). The unstated implication seems to be that Medicare should somehow offload the chronic care portion of the home health benefit.

Ironically, this effort to draw clear distinctions between disability-related and medical needs and, implicitly if not explicitly, to erect a protective fence around home health services that are "legitimately" medical in character is occurring during a time of growing professional consensus about the value of integrating acute, post-acute and supportive services to create systems of care that are flexible, "seamless" and "user-friendly" (Benjamin, 1993; Bishop & Skwara, 1993). Such broadly integrated systems would obviate the need to make distinctions which "are sensible in the abstract, but less and less meaningful in practice, as many beneficiaries require both types of service" (Vladeck & Miller, 1994, p. 9).

Whether the Medicare program is the most appropriate vehicle for financing and providing long-term care at home and, if so, how that care should be configured and coordinated with services covered by Medicaid and other funding streams is a subject that merits thoughtful deliberation and vigorous debate. It is also a subject that raises profound and politically sensitive questions about the division of responsibilities between public and private entities, the federal government and the states, payers and providers, and formal and informal caregivers. It is not at all clear that Congress is prepared to frontally attack those questions or to take on fundamental long-term care reform, particularly in the aftermath of the Clinton health care plan. Moreover, popular preferences notwithstanding, politicians and policy makers have shown longstanding reluctance to expand public financing for chronic care at home through explicit policy mandates (Benjamin, 1993). Thus advocates for the elderly and disabled, along with home health industry interests and states that are currently shifting part of their chronic care burden to Medicare home health, may be reluctant to push the issue.

In the near term, then, it seems likely that Congress and the administration will pursue a course of relatively modest incremental reform, designed to alleviate immediate budgetary pressures on the Part A Trust Fund and to allow the home health benefit to evolve over time. What incremental policies can be pursued to improve the efficiency of home health services and constrain the growth of Medicare spending while addressing the needs of beneficiaries for both post-acute and chronic care? Without presuming to speak for the home health research community, it is probably safe to assert that three incremental strategies are consistent with the existing knowledge base.

The first is payment reform designed to move away from fee-for-service "piece work" incentives. Just as the policy, practice, and research communities forged consensus around the need to replace retrospective cost-based reimbursement for hospitals with a prospective payment system, so the respective communities in the home health arena are developing consensus around some form of prospective payment for Medicare home health. Virtually everyone involved in the analysis or delivery of home health care would agree that the current cost-based per visit reimbursement system has several undesirable attributes:

1) It rewards providers for delivering additional units of service irrespective of their marginal benefits or costs;
2) It deters innovative efforts to substitute cost-effective alternatives such as telemonitoring, personal emergency response systems, or assistive devices for some portion of in-home visits;
3) It detracts from efforts to focus on the patient or the episode of care, rather than on a discrete encounter; and
4) It is not well suited to outcomes measurement or reporting (Vladeck & Miller, 1994). The Balanced Budget Act of 1997 (PL 105-33) mandated that in fiscal year 2000, HCFA start implementing some form of prospective payment system.[6] While the precise dimensions of home health payment reform have yet to be determined, HCFA's current development work suggests that per-episode payment is a likely candidate. Because per-episode payment creates strong incentives to reduce both costs per visit and visits per episode, a valid case-mix adjuster is necessary to protect service access for individuals with complex and costly conditions and to deter profit-maximizing agencies from "skimming" less difficult cases (Schlenker & Shaughnessy, 1992).

A second incremental strategy that would both build on and reinforce the existing knowledge base is continued testing and evaluation of new models of care within both fully and partially integrated service systems. HCFA is already devoting significant resources to learning from three major demonstrations with different degrees of service integration. The PACE model (Program of All-Inclusive Care for the Elderly) is a fully integrated capitated system that combines Medicare and Medicaid funding

---

[6]The Balanced Budget Act also established an "Interim Payment System" (IPS) intended to cap home health spending during the period 1998 and 1999, before prospective payment is adopted. The IPS imposes an annual per beneficiary limit based on 1993 utilization and costs. The per beneficiary limit is derived by dividing 1993 costs (adjusted for inflation) by the number of unduplicated beneficiaries served in 1993. That per beneficiary limit is then multiplied by the number of unduplicated beneficiaries served in 1998 or 1999 to determine an aggregate limit for the respective year. The limit allows agencies to balance the costs of higher cost versus lower cost patients. Nevertheless it is likely to discourage the provision of service to beneficiaries with long lengths of stay and/or very high service needs.

streams for nursing-home eligible individuals and covers all acute, post-acute, and long-term care. PACE eliminates the perverse incentives embodied in fragmented, fee-for-service categorical programs and based on the experience of its precursor, the San Francisco OnLok program, shows great promise of cost-effectiveness. So far, however, the replication sites have failed to attract large numbers of enrollees (Branch, Coulan, & Zimmerman, 1995). Thus it is possible that PACE will have relatively limited applicability in the armamentarium of home and community-based service reform, even though the Balanced Budget Act facilitates its replication by converting the model from a demonstration project to a permanent benefit category eligible for Medicare coverage and reimbursement.

Somewhat less comprehensive than PACE, the S/HMO (Social Health Maintenance Organization) model integrates acute, post-acute, and some long-term care (about $6500–$12,000 annually)—also under a capitated payment system. Grafted onto established health maintenance organizations, the S/HMO model offers greater promise than PACE for broad-based enrollment. Early evaluation findings, however, suggest that the "first generation" S/HMOs were not successful in producing outcomes superior to those in fee-for-service on mortality, active life expectancy, or health expenditures, despite the availability of chronic care benefits and case management (Newcomer, Harrington, & Manton, 1995; Newcomer, Manton, Harrington, et al., 1995). A second generation of S/HMOs, designed by HCFA to overcome some of the apparent defects of the first generation (including too low a capitation rate, restrictions on enrollment by disability level, and unclear expectations about developing truly geriatrically oriented services), is currently undergoing evaluation (Kane, Kane, & Finch, 1995).

The CNO (Community Nursing Organization) model is the least integrated of the three in that it covers and capitates a partial service package of Medicare home health care and certain Part B ambulatory services, combined with nurse case management. It is the least well known and the least studied of the models to date (the first evaluation findings had not been published at the time of this writing). It is also the model that could be replicated most easily within the existing Medicare home health delivery system. It is therefore well worth watching and replicating, should early results show promise.

While PACE, S/HMOs, and CNOs fall solidly within the movement toward integrated models of care that focus on the beneficiary instead of the unit of service, they are likely to be at best a partial answer to overcoming the fragmentation and perverse incentives of categorical programs and priorities. Also worth supporting and evaluating are other formal demonstrations with varying degrees of integration (e.g., state-sponsored capitated programs for Medicaid long-term care), as well as naturally occurring, market-driven collaborations involving Medicare managed care plans, integrated health systems, and/or home care agencies. As managed care organizations intensify their efforts to enroll Medicare beneficiaries and discover that they are neither experienced, equipped, nor inclined to manage the portion of these enrollees with a complicated mix of medical and supportive service needs, some are turning to home health providers (as well as to so-called "disease state management" companies) to manage for them. It will become increasingly important, therefore, to facilitate and assess cooperative patient management and risk-sharing arrangements between entities that have traditionally managed acute/primary care and those whose expertise is preventive maintenance and ongoing chronic disease management at home and in the community.

The third incremental strategy, which like the second involves the acquisition and analysis of data, calls for uniform and consistent patient assessment and reporting so that the person-level impacts of changes in service delivery and payment can be monitored and evaluated. Congress has already mandated and HCFA has already implemented a uniform minimum data set (MDS) for nursing home residents, which has been used to foster constructive practice changes and quality improvements within the nursing home industry.[7] HCFA is currently supporting the demonstration of OASIS (Outcomes and Assessment Information Set), a core set of data items to be used for outcomes measurement and case-mix adjustment in the home health industry (Shaughnessy, Crisler, & Schlenker, 1995). Like the MDS, the OASIS, if implemented nationally, could support the development, implementation, and refinement of an outcome-based quality improvement system critical for monitoring the patient-level impacts of any new home health payment scheme (Schlenker, 1996). Given that the MDS and the OASIS are geared toward similar patient populations, it is not surprising that they display great similarity in the domains they encompass and the measures they use. Nevertheless, the instruments are sufficiently different to deter easy comparisons between individuals measured by one versus the other. HCFA should therefore place high priority on developing a crosswalk between the two and, ideally, forging them into a single set of measures that would facilitate comparisons between individuals in the institutional and community-care sectors. Moreover, given the high level of interest in comprehensive integrated delivery and payment systems, it would seem sensible to explore

---

[7]Despite the apparent usefulness of the MDS, in a burst of "deregulation" Congress voted to eliminate mandated reporting in the budget bill of 1995 that was vetoed by President Clinton.

the possibility of developing a single instrument that, perhaps in modular form, could be used to assess patients and track outcomes across the full continuum of acute, post-acute and long-term care.

Over the long run, depending on how political and market forces play out, it is possible that the Medicare home health program and along with it the home health industry could be bifurcated and dismantled, with post-acute care absorbed by managed care organizations or integrated hospital systems and long-term care devolved to community-based organizations with a less pronounced medical orientation. Alternatively, it is possible that home health agencies, ideally situated to build bridges between managed care on the one hand and social welfare agencies on the other, could become the hub of community nursing and chronic care activities that successfully integrate both medical and supportive services. Whether one of these scenarios prevails, or other configurations of payment and service delivery emerge, all of these hold the potential to produce either harm or benefit for real people in real time. For that reason it is critical to develop and nurture the system's capacity to monitor and make valid comparisons of cost, quality, and patient outcomes across multiple and varied geographical areas and service settings.

REFERENCES

Benjamin, A. E. (1986). Determinants of state variations in home health utilization and expenditures under Medicare. *Medical Care, 24,* 535–547.

Benjamin, A. E. (1993). An historical perspective on home care policy. *Milbank Quarterly, 71,* 129–166.

Bishop, C. E., & Katon, S. L. (1989). The composition of home health care expenditure growth. *Home Health Care Services Quarterly, 10,* 139–175.

Bishop, C. E., & Skwara, K. C. (1993). Recent growth of medicare home health. *Health Affairs, 12,* 95–110.

Bishop, C. E., Skwara, K. C., & Sangl, J. (1995). *Medicare home health: Expenditure growth and cost-containment potential.* Waltham, MA: Brandeis University. Unpublished manuscript.

Branch, L., Coulan, R., & Zimmerman, Y. (1995). The PACE evaluation: Initial findings. *The Gerontologist, 35,* 349–359.

Cohen, M., & Tumlinson, A. (1997). Understanding the state variation in Medicare home health care: The impact of Medicaid program characteristics, state policy and provider attributes. *Medical Care, 35,* 618–633.

Congressional Research Service. (1996). *Medicare's home health benefit.* (CRS Report for Congress). Washington, DC: Author. (95-1009 EPW).

Duggan v Bowen, (1988). U.S. District Court for the District of Columbia, Number 87-0383, August 1, 1988.

Goldberg, H., & Schmitz, R. (1994). Contemplating home health PPS: Current patterns of Medicare service use. *Health Care Financing Review, 16,* 109–130.

Hastings Center Report. The technological tether: An introduction to ethical and social issues in high-tech home care. Briarcliff Manor, New York: *Hastings Center Special Supplement,* Sept.–Oct. 1994.

HCFA Bureau of Data Management & Strategy. (1995). *Persons using home health agency services, visits, total charges, and program payments, by number of visits: Calendar years 1987 and 1994.* Unpublished manuscript.

HCFR Medicare & Medicaid Statistical Supplement. (1995). *Trends in Medicare home health agency utilization and payment: CYs 1974–93.* Baltimore, MD: U.S. Department of Health & Human Services.

Hedrick, S., & Inui, T. (1986). The effectiveness and cost of home care: An information synthesis. *Health Services Research, 20,* 851–880.

Helbing, C., Sangl, J., & Silverman, H. (1992). Home health agency benefits. *Health Care Financing Review: Annual Supplement,* 125–148.

Hughes, S. (1985). Apples and oranges? A review of evaluations of community-based long-term care. *Health Services Research, 20,* 461–488.

Hughes, S., Cummings, M., Weaver, F., Manheim, L., Conrad, K., & Nash, K. (1990). A randomized trial of Veterans Administration home care for severely disabled veterans. *Medical Care, 28,* 135–145.

Hughes, S. L., Ulasevich, A., Weaver, F., Henderson, W., Manheim, L., Kubal, J., & Bonarigo, F. (1997). Impact of home care on hospital days: A meta-analysis. *Health Services Research, 32,* 415–432.

Kane, R. L., Finch, M., Blewett, L., Burns, R., & Maskowitz, M. (1994). Post-hospital home health care for Medicare patients. *Health Care Financing Review, 16,* 131–155.

Kane, R. L., & Kane, R. A. (1987). *Long-term care: Principles, programs, and policies.* New York: Springer Publishing Co.

Kane, R. L., Kane, R. A., & Finch, M. (1995). Once and future SHMOs. *The Gerontologist, 35,* 294–295.

Kane, R. L., Kane, R. A., Ladd, R. C., & Nielsen, W. (1995). *Variation in state Medicaid spending for long-term care.* Washington, DC: U.S. Department of Health and Human Services, Administration on Aging for the University's National information Sharing Program on Home and Community-Based Services.

Kemper, P. (1988). The evaluation of the National Long-Term Care Demonstration: 10. Overview of the findings. *Health Services Research, 23,* 161–174.

Kenney, G., Coughlin, T., & Rimes, C. (1995, June 6). *The use of Medicare and Medicaid home health services among the joint beneficiary population.* Paper presented at the 12th Annual Meeting of the Association for Health Services Research, Chicago, IL.

Kenney, G., & Dubay, L. (1992). Explaining area variation in the use of Medicare home health services. *Medical Care, 30,* 43–57.

Liu, K., McBride, T. D., & Coughlin, T. A. (1990). Costs of community care for disabled elderly persons: The policy implications. *Inquiry, 27,* 61–72.

Long, S. (1994). *Caring for the frail elderly: Does formal care substitute for informal care?* Washington, DC: Urban Institute. Unpublished manuscript.

Manton, K., Corder, L., & Stallard, E. (1993). Estimates of change in chronic disability and institutional incidence and prevalence rates in the U.S. elderly population from 1982, 1984 and 1989 National Long-Term Care Survey. *Journals of Gerontology: Social Sciences, 48,* S153–S166.

Manton, K., Stallard, E., & Woodbury, M. (1994). Home health and skilled nursing facility use: 1982–90. *Health Care Financing Review, 16,* 155–186.

Mauser, E. (1995, October–November). *Does organizational form matter: Implications for the home health industry.* Paper presented at the American Public Health Association Meetings, San Diego, CA.

Mauser, E. (1996). *Distribution of home health users across visit categories: Users with more and less than 150 visits in 1992: Data from the Medicare Beneficiary Survey, 1992.* Unpublished manuscript.

Mauser, E., & Miller, N. A. (1994). A profile of home health users in 1992. *Health Care Financing Review, 16,* 17–33.

Mauser, E., & Miller, N. A. (1995, June 6). The growth of hospital-based home health agencies: Vertical integration as strategic behavior. Paper presented at the 12th Annual Meeting of the Association for Health Services Research, Chicago, IL.

Mehlman, M. J., & Youngner, S. J. (1991). *Delivering high technology home care.* New York: Springer Publishing Co.

Miller, N., Mauser, E., & Harrington, C. (1995, October 30–November 2). *Explaining variation in Medicaid community-based long-term care expenditures: 1987–1993.* Paper presented at the American Public Health Association Meeting, San Diego, CA. Baltimore, MD: HCFA, ORD. Unpublished.

Newcomer, R. J., Harrington, C., Manton, K. G., & Lynch, M. (1995). A response to representatives from the social HMOs regarding program evaluation. *The Gerontologist, 35,* 292–293.

Newcomer, R. J., Manton, K. G., Harrington, C., Yordi, C., & Vertrees, J. (1995). Case-mix controlled service use and expenditures in the Social/Health Maintenance Organization demonstration. *Journal of Gerontology: Medical Sciences, 50A,* M35—M44.

Office of Inspector General. (1995). *Geographical variation in visits provided by home health agencies* (OEI-04-93-00262). Washington, DC: Department of Health and Human Services.

Prospective Payment Commission (1996, March). *Report and recommendations to the Congress.* Washington, DC: Author.

Prospective Payment Commission (1997, June). *Medicare and the American health care system: Report and recommendations to the Congress.* Washington, DC: Author.

Rich, M., Beckham, V., Wittenberg, C., Leven, C., Freedland, K., & Carney, R. (1995). A multidisciplinary intervention to prevent the readmission of elderly patients with congestive heart failure. *New England Journal of Medicine, 333,* 1190–1195.

Richardson, S., Huang, A., Podsiado, D., & Gayton, D. (1995). Geriatric day hospitals. *JAGS, 43*(10), 1179–1181.

Schlenker, R. (1996). *Home health payment legislation: Review and recommendations* (Public Policy Institute #9611). Washington, DC: American Association of Retired Persons.

Schlenker, R., & Shaughnessy, P. (1992). Medicare home health reimbursement alternatives: Access, quality and cost incentives. *Home Health Care Services Quarterly, 13*, 91–115.

Schore, J. (1994, September 30). Patient, agency, and area characteristics associated with regional variation in the use of Medicare home health services. Princeton, NJ: Mathematica Policy Research Inc. Unpublished.

Shaughnessy, P. W., Crisler, K., & Schlenker, R. (1995). Measuring and assuring the quality of home health care. *Health Care Financing Review, 16*, 35–68.

Shaughnessy, P. W., Schlenker, R. E., & Hittle, D. F. (1994). Home health care outcomes under capitated and fee-for-service payment. *Health Care Financing Review, 16*, 187–222.

Silverman, H. (1990). Use of Medicare-covered home health agency services, 1988. *Health Care Financing Review, 12*, 113–126.

Stuck, A., Aronow, H., Steiner, A., Alessi, C., Bula, C., Gold, M., Yuhas, K., Nisenbaum, R., Rubenstein, L., & Beck, J. (1995). A trial of annual in-home comprehensive geriatric assessments for elderly people living in the community. *New England Journal of Medicine, 333*, 1184–1189.

Swan, J. H., & Benjamin, A. E. (1992). Medicare home health utilization as a function of nursing home market factors. *Health Services Research, 25*, 479–500.

U.S. General Accounting Office. (1990). *Medicare: Increased denials of home health claims during 1986 and 1987* (B-225004). Washington, DC: Author.

U.S. General Accounting Office. (1996). *Medicare: Home health utilization expands while program controls deteriorate* (GAO/HEHS-96-16). Washington, DC: Author.

Vladeck, B., & Miller, N. (1994). The Medicare home health initiative. *Health Care Financing Review, 16*, 7–16.

Weissert, W. (1991). A new policy agenda for home care. *Health Affairs, 10*, 67–77.

Weissert, W., Cready, C., & Pawelak, J. (1988). The past and future of home and community-based long-term care. *Milbank Quarterly, 66*, 309–388.

Weissert, W., & Hedrick, S. (1994). Lessons learned from research on effects of community-based long-term care. *Journal of the American Geriatrics Society, 42*, 348–353.

Weissert, W., Wan, T., Livierqators, B., & Pellegrino, J. (1980). Cost-effectiveness of homemaker services for the chronically ill. *Inquiry, 17*, 230–243.

Welch, H. G., Wennberg, D., & Welch, W. P. (1996). The use of Medicare home health care services. *New England Journal of Medicine, 335*, 324–329.

Williams, B. (1994). Comparison of services among different types of home health agencies. *Medical Care, 32*, 1134–1152.

4
The Geriatric Day Hospital

Lois K. Evans
Mary Ann Forciea
Johanna Yurkow
Julie Sochalski

INTRODUCTION

Simultaneous accelerations in both the aging of America and the profound transformation in the health care system, together with demographic changes affecting family caregiving, make imperative a consideration of a range of community-based daytime care options. The frail elderly, suffering from complex physical, emotional, and cognitive problems, often find themselves the casualties of a health care delivery system that focuses on curative, rather than restorative, interventions. Few alternatives may be available through the continuum of care from acute hospitalization to long-term placement (Densen, 1991). From a humanitarian as well as a cost-containment perspective, long-term care for the elderly suffering with chronic diseases has become a significant societal problem (Kunz & Shannon, 1996). It has become essential that the continuum of care for the frail elderly be expanded to include more home, community-based, and transitional services. These services should be directed at sustaining the elder, following a period of decline or cascading event, in independent or supportive living at an optimal level of functioning. An individualized approach is imperative.

Among the several day service models in existence, only the geriatric day hospital provides the level of comprehensive assessment, diagnostic, and treatment (including rehabilitation) options likely to impact utilization of institutional or ambulatory clinical resources. Of European origin, the geriatric day hospital (GDH) has a long history, yet little convincing empiric evidence exists for its greater cost-benefit in providing care for frail elders. A re-examination of the evidence is important if the GDH is to play a role in the evolving managed care environment in which risk is shared among insurer and provider/systems. In this chapter we briefly review a range of community-based models for older adults, describe the history and development of the geriatric day hospital together with relevant outcomes-related research, and describe one model for day hospital services in a case study. Suggestions for future study are made.

COMMUNITY-BASED MODELS OF CARE FOR FRAIL ELDERS

There currently exist many models of community-based care for frail elders which share, at least in the broadest context, similar goals. These include improving or maintaining community integration and feelings of well-being, improving skills that promote independent living, and minimizing time spent in an institutional setting (Sherwood, Morris, & Ruchlin, 1986). Labels for these services are often used interchangeably to describe a spectrum of services, making comparison between and among program types difficult at best. A "senior center" may consist merely of a nutrition site for older adults or a multiservice agency providing a broad range of social and health services. Likewise, the term "day hospital" is applied in the literature to medical day care, adult day health care, and partial (mental) hospital services. Such confusion in labelling, among other issues, has severely curtailed the ability to evaluate differential outcomes of the various types of community-based services or to knowledgeably interpret findings of published research. For example, Sherwood et al. (1986) claim to have compared quality-of-life outcomes among a range of long-term care options, including the "day hospital" [closer to "medical day care" than day hospital], senior centers (a full range of types), and nursing home (a mixture of both skilled and intermediate facilities), finding no major differences in quality-of-life effects for the three options after 9 months of placement! The major types of community-based options will each be defined and briefly described before turning to the day hospital.

Senior Center Programs

Multiservice senior centers are primarily social organizations organized around a nutritional program, including at least a hot meal at midday, and a range of social and recreational programs (Sherwood et al., 1986). Often transportation to medical appointments and shopping, advocacy counseling, education, and information and referral services are also offered. Generally, older adults who attend senior centers are less functionally impaired than are those utilizing other community programs. Direct health services, other than health information and promotion, are not usually provided. Programming for senior centers derives from the Administration on Aging through Area Agencies on Aging.

Adult Day Care

The psychosocial model of adult day care (ADC) has its roots in dementia care; in Great Britain, ADC is termed the "day centre." While socialization and recreational activities are included, often in an individualized program which may include some custodial care, a major rationale for ADC is caregiver respite. Today's ADCs may be dementia-specific, dementia nonspecific, or nondementia type, depending on the proportional inclusion of persons with dementia (Cefalu, Ettinger, & Espeland, 1996). Many ADC centers are unable to care for elders who present with certain behaviors, e.g., aggression, wandering, incontinence, or severe functional limitations, and are thus limited in their ability to delay institution-based care. Depending on the type of services offered, payment may come from out-of-pocket or Medicaid (through waiver programs), with Administration on Aging funds helping to subsidize ADC care in many communities ("How states use Medicaid waivers," 1994).

Adult Day Health Care/Medical Day Care

Termed the "health model" of adult day care, medical or adult day health care (ADHC) is a "therapeutically oriented ambulatory day program which provides health maintenance and rehabilitative services to frail elderly individuals in a congregate setting during daytime hours" (Connis et al., 1993, p. SS26). In addition to recreation, meals, transportation, counseling and information/referral services, assessment and monitoring by a health care provider, and access to restorative/maintenance rehabilitative services are provided (Sherwood et al., 1986). Such programs are expected to benefit patients through more intensive medical and auxiliary services, including closer supervision and monitoring and more frequent provision of rehabilitative services; family caregivers can also anticipate benefits, both through respite and through improved functioning in the elder for whom they provide care at home (Rothman, Hedrick, Bulcroft, Erdly, & Nickinovitch, 1993). In the Program for All-Inclusive Care for the Elderly (PACE) sites, adult day health care centers form the hub for PACE assessment, monitoring, medical, rehabilitation, and social intervention (Eng, Pedulla, Eleazer, McCann, & Fox, 1997). For PACE enrollees, capitated fees under Medicaid/Medicare waivers cover the cost of ADHC; veteran's fees are paid by the VA; and some insurers pay for selected components of ADHC services, particularly rehabilitation components, while others pay out of pocket.

The Veteran's Administration (VA) has made rather extensive use of this model, both through direct provision and under contract to community facilities, as a substitute for nursing home, hospital, and other health care services (home care, ambulatory care) for chronically ill veterans (Ehreth, Chapko, Hedrick, & Savirono, 1993). A recent extensive evaluation of veteran-utilized ADHCs identified an average length of stay of 199 days [range 0 to 371 days] defined as number of days between patient's first and last visits (Connis et al., 1993). Overall, patients receiving ADHC reported greater satisfaction with their care than did those receiving either nursing home or home care, but neither they nor their caregivers reported any differences in health outcomes compared with those receiving customary care (Rothman et al., 1993). Only three subgroups—those not married, those most satisfied with their social support network, and those not hospitalized at time of study enrollment—had better outcomes on the Sickness Impact Profile. A detailed cost/benefit evaluation of ADHC revealed that veterans who used VA-delivered ADHC services had 15% greater overall healthcare costs on average than did the matched comparison group (Hedrick et al., 1993).

Partial Hospital

The partial hospital (PH) has mental health service system origins, particularly for the seriously mentally ill (Cummings, Kerner, Arones, & Steinbeck, 1985). In Great Britain, the psychogeriatric day hospital is comparable. Since the advent of the community mental health center movement in the U.S., partial hospital programs have provided services either during the day or during the night for persons requiring more support than could be provided in outpatient care, yet at less intense levels than that provided in the hospital setting. More recently, partial hospital programs geared specifically to older adults have evolved. Primarily, these programs provide services to elders residing in nursing homes or in the community who are recovering from depression or other mental disturbances, or target elders with dementia who display behaviors that staff or families find difficult to manage. Partial hospital costs are borne by Medicare, other third-party payors, and consumers.

Geriatric Day Hospital

With origins in Great Britain, geriatric day hospitals (GDH) are aimed at facilitating earlier hospital discharge, preventing readmission, and maintaining community residence for older people requiring extensive medical and rehabilitative services. For Britain's National Health Service, the functions of a GDH are rehabilitation, maintenance, assessment, medical, nursing, and social care (Brockelhurst, 1995). In Canada, the day hospital is seen as an organized program of necessary services provided in a day setting for noninstitutionalized elderly and disabled adults who require diagnostic, rehabilitative, or therapeutic services on a scheduled basis (Greve, 1985). Siu, Morishita, and Blaustein (1994) define the GDH as

> an outpatient facility where frail older patients can receive subacute or acute medical, nursing, social and/or rehabilitative services over any portion of a full day, with return visits as necessary. This definition excludes day hospital programs with more restricted or single purposes (such as rehabilitation, psychiatry, or cancer care only) and programs with a more social/less medical orientation (p. 1094).

Particularly in the UK, geriatric care providers have a strong belief in the superiority of day hospital care for frail elderly, particularly those unable to adequately use a traditional outpatient care system. GDH features of most importance are its extensive use of the multidisciplinary team, individualized plans of treatment, and integration within a geriatric system of services where it can serve as a bridge between hospital and community (Ames & Hastie, 1995). In the U.S., financial reimbursement for GDH services is most often through commercial insurers, at least for the rehabilitation and medical therapy portions; Medicare, for those day hospitals certified as a Comprehensive Outpatient Rehabilitation Facility (CORF); and the Veteran's Administration (Cummings et al., 1985; Evans, Yurkow, & Siegler, 1995; Hedrick et al., 1993).

HISTORY AND EVOLUTION OF THE GERIATRIC DAY HOSPITAL

The development of geriatric services in Great Britain is traced to Dr. Marjorie Warren, who initially described her experiences in the treatment of chronically ill elders in the late 1930s. She pioneered the concept of comprehensive assessment of older institutionalized patients, described multidisciplinary teams of professionals working together to establish goals and treatments for her patients, and published results showing that such careful assessment could result in the discharge of "incurable" older patient back into their communities. Sir Ferguson Anderson extended this comprehensive team evaluation to both the primary care and inpatient settings. By the time the National Health Service (NHS) was created following World War II, not only was the concept of geriatrics well-established as a discipline, but comprehensive team assessment and geriatric rehabilitation guidelines were recognized.

Geriatric Day Hospital in Britain

An integral component of the British system of geriatric care, the model for the geriatric day hospital was developed at Oxford in 1951 to ease the transition between acute hospital stay and care at home. Many day hospitals continue to use the original Oxford physical plant design of a square facility surrounding a central garden, so that even confused patients can be allowed safe access to the outside. Many day hospitals also perpetuate the basic approach of the early units: Patients are referred by primary care physicians or hospital-based specialists; outpatients are transported by the NHS ambulances services at no cost to patients or families; initial comprehensive assessments are performed by team members; and rehabilitation goals are set and regularly reviewed at interdisciplinary team meetings.

The concept of the day hospital has been widely accepted in Great Britain, so that today at least 400 day hospitals are in existence there (Brockelhurst, 1995). The majority of British facilities are based at hospitals, offer physical and occupational therapy, accept both inpatients and outpatients, and serve a geographic catchment area. They operate 5 days a week, although most patients visit only 2 or 3 times per week (Brockelhurst, 1979). Variations on the day hospital theme abound in Britain; some facilities focus on a single area of treatment (the psychogeriatric day hospital, for example) and some offer diagnostic as well as therapeutic services. A continuing point of controversy, however, is the issue of service duration. Most British day hospitals offer time limited (e.g., 1–5 visits/week for up to 12 weeks) attendance, yet many proponents believe that long-term services should be provided (Brockelhurst, 1979). Several UK day hospital programs have been described in the literature (Eagle et al., 1991; Greve, 1985; Martinez, Carpenter, & Williamson, 1984;

Tucker, Davison, & Ogle, 1983), and many of these are acknowledged to have at least a proportion of long-stay or chronic attenders. Another problem in the British system has been a lack of uniformity in basic services, which has made outcome studies difficult (Evans, 1983). The Royal College of Physicians (Brockelhurst, 1995) proposed minimum guidelines for effective day hospital function that would include: A written policy statement of the goals and services of the individual day hospital; a plan of care with clear goals for each patient that are agreed on by the team, patient, and caregiver; adequate staff to allow a key worker to supervise each patient in his plan of care; and regular monitoring of performance and cost.

Geriatric Day Hospital in the U.S.

In the United States, the GDH has its roots in rehabilitation medicine. Following reinvigoration by Howard Rusk's work with injured soldiers after World War II, rehabilitation embraced multidisciplinary functional assessment and individualized goals, with a focus on improvement in functional ability (Torres-Gil & Wray, 1993). In the post-World War II era, rehabilitation became increasingly viewed as a strategy for restoring health and function following trauma or an acute illness such as a spinal cord injury, stroke, or amputation. Such services might be offered after hospitalization, but were less frequently provided for functional limitations created by chronic disease. Most primary care physicians remained uncomfortable with the therapeutic capabilities of rehabilitation therapies and continued to have difficulty with prescribing optimal levels. Few medical schools and primary care residencies offered curricular time to rehabilitation issues. Thus, as compared with the British experience, rehabilitation, especially as it related to the older adult, remained marginalized in the U.S.

Medicare reimbursement for geriatric rehabilitation has served to reinforce the concept of acute illness-based rehabilitation. Medicare Part A is a hospital insurance program which also covers some inpatient rehabilitation care related to recovery from a specific illness. In fact, Medicare regulations require that a patient participate in a minimum of 3 hours per day of structured rehabilitation in order to qualify for inpatient rehabilitation services. Many older patients find such programs too rigorous following an acute illness, and are, thus, ineligible for inpatient rehabilitation. Outpatient rehabilitation is partially covered by Medicare Part B, as long as the therapy is physician-ordered, and as long as the patient is making progress towards a goal. The chronically ill older patient with multisystem disabilities who is struggling to maintain function has often found himself unable to qualify for services (Torres-Gil & Wray, 1993), or unable to be adequately managed in the usual outpatient rehabilitation service.

Successful day hospital programs for younger psychiatric patients first emerged at the Yale and Menninger Clinics in the late 1940s (Cummings et al., 1985). The first U.S. geriatric day hospitals were not established until 1973 at the Burke Rehabilitation Center in White Plains, New York (Lorenz, Hamill, & Oliver, 1974) and the Moss Rehabilitation Hospital in Philadelphia in 1976 (Cummings et al., 1985), more than 20 years later than in the UK. Since then, a slow but steady increase has been seen in the number of geriatric day hospitals in the U.S. Most focus on assessment and short-term diagnostic and treatment goals which can be achieved in 2–3 visits per week over a 6–8 week period.

The convergence of the British and U.S. models of geriatric day hospital care can be seen as a testament to the importance of comprehensive functional assessment and interdisciplinary team care that has become the hallmark of good geriatric care. Further, advances in the recognition of geriatric comprehensive assessment as a tool which leads to better function is beginning to produce reimbursement mechanisms—often a barrier to services in American health care—related to functional assessment in both inpatient and outpatient arenas. Still, in part because the day hospital does not "fit" well with traditional payment streams, its proliferation has not been widespread. Lack of clear scientific evidence in the cost-effectiveness of such programs has also impeded its development.

EVALUATION/MEASUREMENT CHALLENGES

An early study in Britain (Woodford-Williams, McKeon, Trotter, Watson, & Bushby, 1962) revealed that day hospital patients were hospitalized less often and showed improvements in mental and physical health. New Zealand investigators reported that rehabilitation in a day hospital resulted in similar improved outcomes (Tucker et al., 1984). A Canadian study, however, found no significant benefit in functional status or quality of life in GDH patients compared with those receiving usual outpatient care (Eagle et al., 1991). Further, a UK study found that improvement in functional ability was greater in stroke patients randomized to home physiotherapy rather than to day hospital treatment (Young & Forster, 1992). Many problems in the existing day hospital research literature have led to such contradictory and equivocal results and severely limit generalizability. These problems can be categorized in terms of definition, design, measurement, and sample size.

Differences in Definition and Patient Population

Several different types of GDHs and other DHs exist both in the U.S. and other health care systems. Without a clear definition of the model being tested, their experiences are not generalizable. For example, at the GDH at Century City Hospital Center for Geriatric Health, affiliated with the UCLA Department of Medicine, patients receive comprehensive geriatric assessment, close medical monitoring and acute nursing care, multiple diagnostic investigations, and intensive coordinated rehabilitation and case management (Morishita et al., 1989). This GDH is located within a hospital and accesses hospital services for attendees. A recent evaluation indicating poor outcomes (Siu et al., 1994) is found, on closer scrutiny, to have only measured one component (comprehensive geriatric assessment). In day hospital programs for specific populations, e.g. cancer patients, recent evaluations have demonstrated greatly reduced costs for DH patients as compared with inpatient users in a randomized clinical trial; in addition, there were no differences in health and psychosocial outcomes between the two groups (Mor et al., 1988). In this case, substitutive care (day care for 24-hour hospital care) was found to be equivalent in outcomes, but superior in terms of cost-effectiveness. Whether other types of GDH are really providing substitutive care, or care that otherwise would not have been available to a specified population, is an important question. Much like the geriatric evaluation and management (GEM) unit studies, investigators studying day hospital effects are concluding that attention to specific patient populations for whom the day hospital may be most effective or appropriate as well as control over an appropriate interval (dose) of care are essential (Donaldson, Wright, & Maynard, 1986) in achieving outcomes.

Design

Small sample size, single-site evaluations, and inclusion of sites with differing programs and level of organizational maturity contribute to design flaws. In a thoughtful review of the GDH literature, Eagle and colleagues (1987) suggested that a GDH should not be evaluated until after it has become fully functional; they acknowledge, however, that randomization is exceedingly difficult to achieve at that point because of patient and provider resistance and concern for fiscal viability. Further, they indicate that generalizability to other settings from single-site evaluation studies is hazardous at best, especially since each "day hospital" appears to have individual characteristics in structure, function, and client populations. In an evaluation of their own GDH, using an investigator-developed instrument, Eagle et al. (1991) found no difference in quality of life outcomes among elders randomly assigned for treatment to either GDH or geriatric outpatient care over a 12-month period. This finding may also be illustrative of a further limitation in study methods: lack of appropriate instrumentation.

Instrumentation

Selection of appropriate outcome criteria to be measured is imperative; for example, in acutely oriented GDH, improvement in functional status may be sought, whereas in those GDHs serving more long-term care and respite needs, maintenance in functional status and reduction in caregiver burden would seem more appropriate (Brockelhurst, 1995). Brockelhurst notes that in one recent study (1995), where patients were categorized in active and maintenance cohorts, the outcomes were as hoped for, while other controlled trials of day hospital outcomes yielded only equivocal results. Similarly, Siu et al. (1994) found no significant effects of comprehensive assessment in the GDH, compared with clinic sites without a day hospital, on mortality, use of emergency or hospital service, placement, or change on selected measures of health status; whether comprehensive assessment should be assumed to affect these outcomes is in question, especially since the GDH staff had no control over patient compliance with recommendations (Richardson, Hyang, Podsiado, & Gayton, 1995).

Lack of instruments that are sensitive to the more subtle functional changes achieved in outpatient care is also problematic (Cameron, 1993; Evans, Yurkow, & Siegler, 1995; Parker et al., 1993). Many instruments have been normed on inpatients, where more rapid and gross improvements are expected. Potential for the use of methods like goal-attainment scaling to measure clinical outcomes is being addressed (Rockwood, Stolee, & Fox, 1993). Further, it is important to consider, at least for certain types of day hospital programs, the outcome in terms of relief of caregiver burden as well (Donaldson et al., 1986). It would appear that many factors influence elders' selection of/use of long-term care options, including availability and knowledge of certain options (Sherwood et al., 1986).

Cost as an important outcome has yet to be adequately defined in GDH studies (Donaldson et al., 1986). One question is whether cost should include only the operation of the GDH, or also the contributions of the family and other services, such as home help, home nursing, and day care, that have helped to maintain the elder in the community. If the day hospital is not a separate cost center but shares services and personnel with, for example, an inpatient unit, determining actual cost per patient day is difficult as is estimating the cost of ambulance or other transportation services, especially when these are subsidized. For how long a period should cost and outcomes be measured? Many studies follow patients over periods from 3 months to 1 year post-discharge, but most have no results after the 5-week or 3-month period, indicating perhaps that results are not sustained. Donaldson and colleagues (1986) recommend that the following outcomes be measured: cost of service utilization per patient during and subsequent to GHD use; clinical, social, and psychological outcome data for each subgroup before, during and at the end of the study period, plus a measure of patient and caregiver satisfaction.

THE CARE PROGRAM: A CASE EXAMPLE

The Collaborative Assessment and Rehabilitation for Elders (CARE) Program is an academic practice of the University of Pennsylvania School of Nursing (SON), operated in collaboration with the School of Medicine (SOM) and the University of Pennsylvania Health System (UPHS). A certified Medicare Comprehensive Outpatient Rehabilitation Facility (CORF), the CARE Program was conceived as an important link between hospital and community-based care for an integrated geriatric service of the UPHS and modelled on the British geriatric day hospital. The Program is located in renovated space on the edge of the campus that houses the comprehensive geriatric, psychogeriatric, and gerontologic nursing clinical practices and the academic offices of the University's geriatric faculty. The goals of this nurse-managed, collaborative practice are to maximize independent functioning, promote health, and enhance quality of life for chronically ill, frail older adults in the community. This is accomplished through interdisciplinary team assessment and collaborative interventions developed around an individualized plan of care. Clients are admitted whose needs are largely unmet by the existing health care delivery system.

Clinical services and operations are managed by a master's-prepared gerontologic nurse practitioner (GNP). Clinical staff from three rehabilitation departments at UPHS (physical, occupational, and speech therapy); two departments in the SOM (geriatrics and physiatry); and the SON's Penn Nursing Network form an interdisciplinary team that provides services on a day-to-day basis. A GNP assigned to each client serves as care manager, responsible for coordinating, monitoring, and providing care in close collaboration with other team members, as well as with the medical director and the client's primary care provider (Evans et al., 1995).

The CARE Program was specifically designed for a population that needs extensive comprehensive assessment, intensive interdisciplinary interventions, and physical and emotional support for the client as well as the family. This is a group not currently well-served by existing rehabilitation services. Frailty (normally over age 65), multiple and complex needs, and appropriateness for ambulatory care and community living form the major admission criteria. Hallmarks of the Program include integrated interdisciplinary team assessment and intervention aided by use of a problem classification system (Omaha; Martin & Scheet, 1992); time-limited, individualized program of services; advanced nurse practice clinical leadership, care management, and integrated mental health services; extensive evaluation of outcomes at discharge, 1 and 3 months post-discharge, and a formal evaluation research project in progress. Due to the complex nature of the problems experienced by this population, coordination and collaboration are essential to the client's success. All clinicians are particularly sensitive to problems that may potentially interfere with program success. These barriers are not immediately obvious to providers without preparation in treating the geriatric population and may include cognitive dysfunction, depression, abnormal grief patterns, constipation, inappropriate medication administration, and lack of community support, among others. To be appropriately sensitive, clinical assessment tools that have been designed specifically for older adults or modified to address the special needs of this population are required. Details of the program are described elsewhere (Evans et al., 1995). The remainder of this case example will describe and critique the outcome measures and evaluation processes utilized in the CARE Program. Table 4.1 lists the assessment tools used in the initial evaluation and measure of outcomes.

TABLE 4.1 CARE Program Outcome Measures

History and Physical (Brief)
Hearing Handicap Inventory in the Elderly Screening Questionnaire
Nutrition Screening Initiative
Speech-Language Pathology Screening
Mini-Mental State Exam
Geriatric Depression Scale
Medical Outcome Survey—Short Form (Modified)
Functional Independence Measure
Berg Functional Balance Test
Tinetti Balance/Gait Assessment
One- and Three-Month Follow-Up

MEASURING CLINICAL OUTCOMES

In addition to the general clinical evaluation to determine needs, assessment tools are used that measure areas of function normally expected to show improvement while in the Program, identify potential barriers to successful rehabilitation, or indicate areas of knowledge or skill deficits. The instruments include measures of affect, cognitive function, ADL/IADL function, physical and mental health, and sensory and nutritional status.

Medical, Sensory, and Nutritional Status

A brief history and physical examination and screening tools to evaluate hearing, speech, and nutritional deficits are completed only on admission. The brief history and PE may reveal health problems that can be addressed immediately, affecting the client's success in the Program. The sensory and nutrition screens, however, may identify needs that require long-term interventions, such as referrals to speech-language pathology, audiology, ophthalmology, or dental services; extensive dietary education requiring a long-term change in lifestyle; referral for community services; or referral for full cognitive testing. Because the Program is time-limited, it is difficult to evaluate the outcome of these interventions during the client's stay, but compliance with recommendations is assessed during post-discharge follow up. Recommendations are documented on the client's discharge prescription which lists important self-care activities that are to be continued at home.

Cognitive Status

The Folstein Mini-Mental State Exam (MMSE; Folstein, Folstein, & McHugh, 1975) is a well-known screen for cognitive function with utility in clinical practice as well as in research. The MMSE score is the total number of correct answers in 30. Based on the score, a client can be classified as having no cognitive impairment (24–30); mild cognitive impairment (18–23); or severe cognitive impairment (0–17). Much work has been done to evaluate the influence of demographic and social attributes on the MMSE, including educational level, gender, race/ethnicity and social class; of these, age and education exert the greatest effect (Tombaugh & McIntyre, 1992). These factors are taken into consideration in interpreting the MMSE score in the CARE Program. All clients are screened using the MMSE on admission and, if the score is in the impaired range, again at discharge. The admission score assists the staff in identifying any need for referral to the geropsychiatric clinical nurse specialist (GPCNS) for a more comprehensive cognitive evaluation and possible referral to geriatric psychiatry for a full dementia work-up. The test is also helpful in identifying clients that may need additional interventions to assist with carry-over and retention of information. Common interdisciplinary interventions implemented during the program often have a positive effect on the cognitive functioning of the client. These may include discontinuation of unnecessary medications with side effects affecting cognition; improvement in self-esteem and, thus, a lifting of depression; psychotherapy addressing issues related to role, caregiving, or grief; and relief of pain.

Emotional Status

Depression is the most common functional psychiatric condition of late life. It has been estimated that depressive symptoms occur in approximately 15% of community residents over 65. For those elders with chronic physical conditions, however, the relation between physical health impairment and depression is even stronger (Blixen, Wilkinson, & Schuring, 1994). The Geriatric Depression Scale (GDS; Yesavage, 1986) is a 30-point yes/no screening instrument designed for older adults to identify depressive symptoms. The GDS works well in identifying depression in the physically ill and demented populations. Although the 15-item GDS short-form is available, the full 30-question screen is used in the CARE Program for the additional information it provides to the GPCNS when evaluating the client on referral. The GDS is completed on admission and again, for those scoring in the impaired range, on discharge. It is done as part of the initial evaluation to facilitate early recognition of an individual who may be too depressed to cooperate with program efforts, keep appointments, or in some other way comply with interventions to meet identified goals. A score of 11 or greater indicates a possible depression and triggers a referral to the GPCNS, with possible eventual referral to geriatric psychiatry. In severe cases, the client may be discharged from the program to facilitate geropsychiatric follow-up and allow time to obtain a therapeutic level of an antidepressant medication before readmission. In cases of less severe depression, ongoing psychotherapy is provided in conjunction with rehabilitation efforts. In these situations, the GPCNS monitors the client closely for indication of less than full involvement in program activities. In 4–8 weeks the positive effects of mental health interventions in the form of psychotherapy or education are often obvious. Also, individuals who have responded well to rehabilitation efforts, had the opportunity to develop social connections, or have a reduction in pain and other symptomatology often show an improvement in their GDS score. Sometimes, just getting out of the house a few days a week and being around individuals who are respectful and motivating results in improved mood.

Quality-of-Life Status

A modified version of the Medical Outcomes Study—Short Form (MOS-SF 36) is used to measure general health concepts and quality of life. The modified MOS-SF assesses physical functioning, mental health, health perceptions, and pain on a 30-item survey (Stewart, Hays, & Ware, 1988). The survey remains reliable irregardless of age, level of serious chronic conditions, symptoms of depression, or educational level. It was necessary to revise the tool to eliminate six questions related to physical functioning which are assessed in-depth in other portions of the database. Most activities addressed in the section, i.e., lifting heavy objects, running, participation in sports, bowling, carrying groceries, and walking up-hill far exceeded even recent past abilities of the Program population. The modified MOS-SF is repeated at discharge to measure quality-of-life improvement over the course of the Program.

Functional Status

The measurement of functional status is paramount in any program with restoration of physical functioning as a goal. The CARE Program uses three tools to measure baseline and discharge status related to physical functioning.

1. Functional Independence Measure

The Functional Independence Measure (FIM) assesses self care, sphincter management, mobility, locomotion, communication, and social cognition on a 7-point scale (Center for Functional Assessment Research, 1990). The FIM is a basic measure of severity of disability, rather than impairment, and is performance-oriented. The FIM was developed to be discipline-free and thus works well in an interdisciplinary setting. It is helpful to assign FIM areas to those clinicians who are most knowledgeable about the domain being evaluated; for example, in the CARE Program, nursing evaluates bowel and bladder management, whereas physical therapy evaluates mobility. The total score of complete independence in all domains is 126.

The FIM is most appropriate for inpatient rehabilitation facilities (Dodds, Martin, Stolov, & Deyo, 1993) and is used in the CARE Program for lack of a better measure, even though it does not work well in an outpatient setting. For example, learning to use assistive devices may lower the client's score even though safe function and endurance has improved. Further, endurance and pain are not well captured in this instrument, yet they are important factors affecting function in CARE Program clients. FIM scores vary with certain clinical conditions and should decrease with increasing age or comorbidity (Dodds, Martin, Stolov, & Deyo, 1993). The FIM is completed on admission and discharge from the program. While a change in the FIM is an indicator of benefit of care, its validity and clinical importance is questionable in this highly specialized setting. An outpatient version of the FIM is currently in process of development (personal communication with C. Granger, February 1996).

2. Berg Functional Balance Test

The Berg Functional Balance test is an instrument for rating an individual's ability to maintain balance while performing 14 movements required in everyday living. Sitting, standing, reaching, turning, stance, and transfers are measured on a scale of 0 (can't perform) to 4 (able to complete task safely within time parameters) (Berg, Wood-Dauphinee, Williams, & Maki, 1992). This tool is predictive of actual functional balance; a score of 45, out of a maximum score of 56, is a cut-off point between individuals who are safe in independent ambulation, "non-fallers," and those requiring investigation concerning their need for assistive devices or supervision (Thorbahn & Newton, 1996). There is also found to be a high correlation between balance score, visual deficits, and prior falls. The Berg is completed on admission and results are used to plan care, assess safety, and evaluate the need for an assistive device. On discharge, the test is used as an outcome measure to measure program progress.

3. Tinetti Gait/Balance Assessment

The Tinetti Balance [16 points] and Gait [12 points] Assessment is a 16 question performance-oriented test that, like the Berg, also reflects position changes and gait maneuvers necessary during normal daily activities.

This tool combines the balance section of the evaluation with gait. Gait characteristics can guide neurologic and musculoskeletal evaluations by suggesting the location of abnormalities. By combining the various balance and gait observations, and by having the client perform special maneuvers such as walking fast (which may highlight subtler abnormalities not evident at a slower pace), working hypotheses as to the possible sources of problems can be formulated (Tinetti, 1986). The Tinetti Balance and Gait Assessment is done on admission and discharge for all program clients. On admission the information is used to screen for underlying abnormalities, and to identify possible restorative, preventive, and adaptive measures. On discharge information is used to measure outcomes.

Measurement of Post-Discharge Outcomes

To measure the longer-term maintenance of outcomes, a follow-up survey specific to the CARE Program was developed and is conducted via telephone interview. The survey questions individuals about their current functional status, continued compliance with discharge instructions, status of problems, and service utilization since discharge from the Program. The follow-up survey, on a more general level, touches on most aspects of formalized evaluations completed during the client's admission. Questions concerning perception of health status, need for assistance, and status of all problems identified and addressed during the program are graded in comparison to status at time of discharge.

Formal Evaluation Research

Because of the uniqueness of the CARE Program structure and function, and the problems with random assignment of clients addressed above, investigators at the School of Nursing's Center for Health Services and Policy Research have looked to innovative models for studying overall Program outcomes, particularly those associated with cost savings in the greater healthcare system (Lang, Evans, Jenkins, & Matthews, 1996). For a service like the CARE Program to generate widespread replication [especially in the Medicare managed care marketplace], impact on high-cost Medicare services, i.e. emergency department and acute hospital services, will need to be demonstrated. A large-scale study has recently been funded by the National Center for Nursing Research to generate appropriate comparison groups from existing national datasets in order to study CARE Program outcomes. If effective, this model holds potential for evaluating similar health care services.

CONCLUSION

The GDH has a long history, both in Europe and in the U.S. It has not been subjected to sufficient rigorous evaluation to determine its cost-effectiveness for specific patient populations. Its value in promoting quality of life and independent functioning in the community, however, is lauded by proponents, while its high cost compared to less intensive community-based alternatives is criticized in the absence of an evidence base or strict criteria. Given the advent of widescale transition to Medicare managed care, the GDH could play an important role in the continuum of integrated services for a frail older enrolled population. Alternatively, or it may be that, in the end, the day hospital will not be shown to be neither more cost-effective nor productive of better outcomes than other forms of care; yet, because of the societal value for community-based over institutional care, it will prevail.

REFERENCES

Ames, D., & Hastie, I. R. (1995). Geriatric day hospitals: The future? *Postgraduate Medical Journal, 71,* 60–61.

Berg, K. O., Wood-Dauphinee, S. L., Williams, J. I., & Maki, B. (1992). Measuring balance in the elderly: Validation of an instrument. *Canadian Journal of Public Health, 83,* S7–S11.

Blixen, C. E., Wilkinson, L. K., & Schuring, L. (1994). Depression in an elderly clinical population: Findings from an ambulatory care setting. *Journal of Psychosocial Nursing, 32,* 43–48.

Brockelhurst, J. C. (1979). The development and present status of day hospitals. *Age and Ageing, 8*(Suppl), 76–79.

Brockelhurst, J. C. (1995). Geriatric day hospitals. *Age and Ageing, 24,* 89–90.

Cameron, M. (1993, Spring). *Assessment of patient mobility at a busy day hospital.* Book of abstracts, British Geriatric Society meeting, Glasgow, Scotland.

Cefalu, C. A., Ettinger, W. H., & Espeland, M. (1996). A study of the characteristics of the dementia patients and caregivers in dementia-nonspecific adult day care programs. *Journal of the American Geriatric Society, 44,* 654–659.

The Center for Functional Assessment Research, Uniform Data System for Medical Rehabilitation for UDS Data Management Services, State University of New York at Buffalo, Department of Rehabilitation Medicine. (1990). *Guide for the use of the uniform data set for medical rehabilitation including the Functional Independence Measure (FIM)* (Version 3.1).

Connis, R. T., Hedrick, S. C., Ries, L. M., Erdly, W. W., Ehreth, J. L., & Conrad, K. J. (1993). Adult day health care organizational and program characteristics. *Medical Care, 31,* SS26–SS37.

Cummings, V., Kerner, J. F., Arones, S., & Steinbeck, C. (1985). Day hospital services in rehabilitation medicine: An evaluation. *Archives of Physical Medicine and Rehabilitation, 66,* 86–91.

Densen, P. M. (1991). *Tracing the elderly through the health care system: An update* (AHCPR 91-11). Rockville, MD: Department of Health and Human Services.

Dodds, A., Martin, D. P., Stolov, W. C., & Deyo, R. A. (1993). Validation of the Functional Independence measure and its performance among rehabilitation inpatients. *Archives of Physical Medicine Rehabilitation, 74,* 531–536.

Donaldson, C., Wright, K., & Maynard, A. (1986). Determining value for money in a day hospital care for the elderly. *Age and Ageing, 15,* 1–7.

Eagle, D. J., Guyatt, G., Patterson, C., & Turpie, I. (1987). Day hospitals' cost and effectiveness: A summary. *Gerontologist, 27,* 735–740.

Eagle, J., Guyatt, G. H., Patterson, C., Turpie, I., Sackett, B., & Singer, J. (1991). Effectiveness of a geriatric day hospital. *Canadian Medical Association Journal, 144,* 699–704.

Ehreth, J., Chapko, M., Hedrick, S. C., & Savirono, J. E. (1993). Cost of VA adult day health care programs and their effect on utilization and cost of care. *Medical Care, 31,* SS50–SS61.

Eng, C., Pedulla, J., Eleazer, G. P., McCann, R., & Fox, N. (1997). Program of All-Inclusive Care (PACE): An innovative model of integrated geriatric care and financing. *Journal of the American Geriatric Society, 45,* 223–232.

Evans, J. G. (1983). The appraisal of hospital geriatric services. *Community Medicine, 5,* 242–250.

Evans, L. K., Yurkow, J., & Siegler, E. L. (1995). The CARE Program: A nurse-managed collaborative outpatient program to improve function of frail older people. *Journal of the American Geriatrics Society, 43,* 1155–1160.

Folstein, M. F., Folstein, S. E., & McHugh, P. R. (1975). Mini-Mental State: A practical guide for grading the cognitive state of patients for the clinician. *Journal of Psychiatric Research, 12,* 189–198.

Greve, M. (1985). The geriatric day hospital. *Perspectives, 9,* 8–9.

Hedrick, S. C., Rothman, M. L., Chapko, M., Ehreth, J., Diehr, P., Inui, T. S., Connis, R. T., Grover, P. L., & Kelly, J. R. (1993). Summary and discussion of methods and results of the adult day health care evaluation study. *Medical Care, 31,* SS94–SS103.

How states use Medicaid waivers to pay for adult day care services. (1994). *Adult Day Care Letter.* Wall Township, NJ: Health Resources Publishing.

Kunz, E., & Shannon, K. (1996). PACE: Managed care for the frail elderly. *American Journal of Managed Care, 2,* 301–304.

Lang, N. M., Evans, L. K., Jenkins, M., & Matthews, D. (1996). Administrative, financial and clinical data for an academic nursing practice: A case study of the University of Pennsylvania School of Nursing. In *The power of faculty practice* (pp. 79–100). Washington, DC: American Association of Colleges of Nursing.

Lorenz, E. J., Hamill, C. M., & Oliver, R. C. (1974). The day hospital: An alternative to institutional care. *Journal of the American Geriatrics Society, 22,* 316–320.

Martin, K. S., & Scheet, N. J. (1992). *The Omaha System: Applications for community health nursing.* Philadelphia: Saunders.

Martinez, F. M., Carpenter, A. J., & Williamson, J. (1984). The dynamics of a geriatric day hospital. *Age and Ageing, 13,* 34–41.

Mor, V., Stalker, M. Z., Gralla, R., Scher, H. I., Cimma, C., Park, D., Flaherty, A. M., Kiss, M., Nelson, P., Laliberte, L., Schwartz, R., Marks, P. A., & Oettgen, H. F. (1988). Day hospital as an alternative to inpatient care for cancer patients: A random assignment trial. *Journal of Clinical Epidemiology, 41,* 771–785.

Morishita, L., Siu, A. L., Wang, R. T., Oken, C., Cadogan, M. P., & Schwartzman, L. (1989). Comprehensive geriatric care in a day hospital: A demonstration of the British model in the United States. *Gerontologist, 29,* 336–340

Parker, S. G., Du, X., Goodfellow, J., Broughton, D., Cleary, R., & James, O. F. W. (1993). *Measuring outcomes in elderly patients in a geriatric day hospital.* Book of abstracts, British Geriatric Society Spring Meeting, Glasgow, Scotland.

Rockwood, K., Stolee, P., & Fox R. A. (1993). Use of goal attainment scaling in measuring clinically important change in the frail elderly. *Journal of Clinical Epidemiology, 46,* 1113–1118.

Rothman, M. L., Hedrick, S. C., Bulcroft, K. A., Erdly, W. W., & Nickinovich, D. G. (1993). Effects of VA adult day health care on health outcomes and satisfaction with care. *Medical Care, 31,* SS38–SS49.

Siu, A. L., Morishita, L., & Blaustein, J. (1994). Comprehensive geriatric assessment in a day hospital. *Journal of the American Geriatrics Society, 42,* 1094–1099.

Sherwood, S., Morris, J. N., & Ruchlin, H. S. (1986). Alternative paths to long-term care: Nursing home, geriatric day hospital, senior center, and domiciliary care options. *American Journal of Public Health, 76,* 38–44.

Stewart, A. L., Hays, R. D., & Ware, J. E. (1988). The MOS Short-form General Health Survey: Reliability and validity in a patient population. *Medical Care, 26,* 724–735.

Thorbahn, L., & Newton, R. (1996). Use of the Berg Balance Test to predict falls in elderly persons. *Physical Therapy, 76,* 576–583.

Tinetti, M. E. (1986). Performance-oriented assessment of mobility problems in elderly patients. *Journal of the American Geriatrics Society, 34,* 119–126.

Tombaugh, T. N., & McIntyre, N. J. (1992). The Mini-Mental State examination: A comprehensive review. *Journal of the American Geriatrics Society, 40,* 922–935.

Torres-Gil, Wray (1993). Funding and policies affecting geriatric rehabilitation. *Clinics in Geriatric Rehabilitation, 9*(4), 831–840.

Tucker, M. A., Davison, J. G., & Ogle, S. J. (1983). Day hospital rehabilitation. Effectiveness and cost in the elderly: A randomized controlled trial. *British Medical Journal, 289,* 1209–1212.

Yesavage, J. A. (1986). The use of self-rating depression scales in the elderly. In L. W. Poon (Ed.), *Handbook for clinical memory assessment of older adults* (pp. 213–217). Washington, DC: American Psychological Association.

Woodford-Williams, E., McKeon, J. A., Trotter, I. S., Watson, D., & Bushby, C. (1962). The day hospital in the community care of the elderly. *Gerontology Clinic, 4,* 241–256.

Young, J. B., & Forster, A. (1992). The Bradford community stroke trial; Results at six months. *BMJ, 304,* 1085–1089.

5
The PACE Model (Program for All Inclusive Care of the Elderly): A Review

Paul Eleazer
Marsha Fretwell

INTRODUCTION

As the Congress of the United States attempts to both reduce the budget deficit and lower taxes, the two sources of public funds supporting acute and long-term health-care service for the poor, disabled, and aging populations are under intensive scrutiny. Cost-containment efforts in the Medicare program propose to create strong financial incentives for older adults to move into managed-care systems receiving capitated payments. Those efforts in the Medicaid program propose to give the states fixed or capped amounts of money compelling them to design more cost-effective community-based programs for the poor, disabled, and those requiring long-term nursing home care.

While this proposed reduction in the funding of acute and long-term care is producing tremendous anxiety in traditional providers of these services, it is important to note that there are already alternative provider models, operating on a small scale, which have demonstrated the possibility of reducing the costs of acute and long-term care for frail older adults without sacrificing the quality of that care. The PACE (Program for All Inclusive Care of the Elderly) model is a managed-care system that integrates acute and long-term care, inpatient and outpatient care, while also integrating Medicare and Medicaid financing to provide cost-effective care to its frail elderly participants.

This chapter reviews the historical background of OnLok and the PACE model, describes the model of care, discusses the variety of evaluative and quality improvement efforts undertaken by PACE, compares the cost of care in the PACE model with that of other models, and, following a description of the limitations of the model, outlines the future direction of the PACE model in our rapidly evolving health-care system.

HISTORY OF ONLOK AND THE PACE MODEL

Thirty years ago, a group of concerned citizens from the Chinatown/North Beach/Polk Gulch district in San Francisco recognized, with the aging of individuals in their community, a growing need for additional long-term care services. Initially the group planned to build a nursing home and hired a consultant, Marie-Louise Ansak, to study the feasibility of their plan. Based on her background in social work and her knowledge of Great Britain's community geriatric-care systems, Ansak proposed instead that they develop a community-based system of care that relied on outpatient services as well as adult day health care. The first day health center opened in March 1973. The program was called OnLok, which means "peaceful, happy abode."

The first phase in the development of the program focused on the adult day health center, where the frail older participants received meals, personal-care services, and recreational activities as well as nursing, social, and transportation services. The professionals involved in these services developed an interdisciplinary team approach that facilitated the coordination of all of these services. Critical to the success of such a large effort to coordinate diverse services for such a frail group of individuals was the development of a common goal or philosophy of care for the interdisciplinary team and the overall program. The philosophy of the program has been since its inception to maintain the participants of the program in their own community for as long as it is medically, socially, and economically feasible (Shen & Iverson, 1992).

From 1973 to 1978, medical care was provided by the participants' own physicians and/or multiple other specialist physicians, with the OnLok interdisciplinary team attempting to ensure continuity of care through close communication and follow-up with these physicians. By 1978, it was clear, given the significant differences in the philosophy of care between the interdisciplinary team (the biopsychosocial model) and the community physicians (the medical model), that the resulting fragmentation of care was not beneficial to the frail population that OnLok was serving. Therefore, in 1978, the program added its own primary medical care system to the model. This primary-care model included both inpatient and outpatient services and blurred the line between acute and long-term care. The result was improved integration and continuity of care and a perception of improved quality. Recruitment and hiring of the primary-care physicians in the program was based on the physicians' commitment to the shared philosophy of care. They are salaried by the program and participate fully in the interdisciplinary team process of managing care.

The second phase of development of the program occurred between 1978 and 1982, during which time OnLok was awarded a 4-year research and demonstration grant by the Office of Human Development Services and the Administration on Aging (Eng, 1987). The goal of the grant was to develop and implement a consolidated model in which multiple services were coordinated and provided by a single agency, the OnLok interdisciplinary team. In the first 2 years, an additional day health center, primary medical care, and inpatient medical services were integrated into the program, making continuity of care a reality. Financing was provided through Medicare and Medi-Cal, with some private copayment. For one capitated rate, OnLok was responsible for providing all inpatient and outpatient medical care as well as social services, pharmaceuticals, sub-specialty medical care, rehabilitation services, durable medical equipment, and home health care (Ansak, 1990). The model also developed assisted-living housing and transitional housing, which provided further support for the goal of care: maintaining individuals in the community as long as is feasible.

The third phase in the development of the program occurred in 1983 when, by default, OnLok began to assume full financial risk. While Medicare was willing to share risk with Medicaid, California's Department of Health Services was not. Without DHS, Medicare would not participate with OnLok in sharing the risk. OnLok was unable to obtain private reinsurance because there was insufficient actuarial data for long-term care costs. OnLok set up its own reserve fund by setting aside 5% of monthly revenues and by 1989 had funds equaling 2 months' operating costs set aside. In 1985, Congress made OnLok's financing and service demonstration a permanent program, allowing its waivers to remain in effect as long as the program operated successfully.

The fourth phase in the development of this innovative model for delivering acute and long-term care to the frail elderly in their own community began in 1986 with the following question: Are there certain demographic and cultural characteristics of the OnLok model that would prevent it from being generalized throughout the United States? To answer this question, the replication model of OnLok, named PACE, or Program for All Inclusive Care of the Elderly, was initiated in 1986. Grant funding from the Robert Wood Johnson Foundation and other foundations provided resources for program start-ups, and Congress passed legislation that provided waivers for 10 nonprofit community-based organizations throughout the United States to provide comprehensive health care services under Medicare and Medicaid capitation financing. Since that date, ten active PACE sites have been developed and eight have completed the developmental process and are operating under full financial risk: East Boston, MA; Portland, OR; Milwaukee, WI; Columbia, SC; the Bronx, NY; Rochester, NY; El Paso, TX; Denver, CO. The PACE model currently serves approximately 2700 frail older adults from multiple ethnic backgrounds located in geographically diverse communities throughout the United States.

DESCRIPTION OF THE PACE MODEL

The philosophy of the clinical program is to maintain participants in their own community for as long as it is medically, socially, and economically feasible. To achieve this, the PACE model employs four major strategies:

- Targeting the frail older adult exclusively;
- Offering the full spectrum of acute- and long-term care services;
- Integrating care through an interdisciplinary team of service providers; and
- Financing the care through integration of Medicaid, Medicare, and private funds into a single capitation rate, with the provider at financial risk.

Targeting: The Selection Process

The target population for PACE is restricted to individuals who meet all of the following criteria: (1) over age 55, (2) certified for nursing home placement, and (3) residing in a defined geographical area.

Participants are referred to the PACE sites from a variety of sources. Several, but not all, of the sites depend upon referrals from their sponsoring organization. For instance, East Boston depends on referrals from the East Boston Neighborhood Health Center, the Bronx relies on the Beth Abraham Hospital, and Rochester relies on the Rochester General Hospital. In contrast, Portland is more dependent on referrals from Oregon Aging Services Division and adult foster homes than from its sponsoring hospital, and Columbia receives more referrals from families and home health agencies than its hospital (Branch, Coulam, & Zimmerman, 1995).

The intake process involves several steps: an initial telephone screening, a series of home visits to provide prospective enrollees with information about the program and to collect assessment data, the development of a profile of the potential client for presentation to the interdisciplinary team, a series of visits to the adult day health centers to provide information for the potential client and allow assessment by the various team members, and finally a decision by the full interdisciplinary team for acceptance or denial to the program.

Certain client characteristics have been recognized among the PACE models as predictive of the potential success or failure of a client in the clinical programs (Branch et al., 1995). The most important characteristics encouraging acceptance of a candidate include sociability, transport safety, and family support. Characteristics that support denial include severe cognitive impairment (end-stage dementia), disruptive behavior, and substance abuse. Appropriate targeting is central to the function of the model.

Integrated Acute and Long-Term Care

The PACE model incorporates all aspects of health-care services: prevention, primary and specialty care, hospitalization for acute care, rehabilitation services, and long-term care. Table 5.1 describes the acute- and long-term care services provided to PACE enrollees. Thus, all traditional Medicare and Medicaid covered services as well as nontraditional services, such as prevention services, meals, transportation, and friendly visiting, are provided. Because of the philosophy of the program and the assumption of full financial risk by each of the PACE sites, the major thrust of service provision is aimed at prevention of acute illnesses and functional impairments and the treatment of the same in the community as opposed to the acute-care hospital or the nursing home.

In the fully capitated sites in 1995, hospital days averaged 2,399 per 1,000 frail enrollees per year versus an estimated 2,448 days for the general Medicare population (which includes mostly well elderly) in 1994 (Kunz & Shannon, 1996). The average length of stay was 4.77 days, and nursing home days represented 6% of total capitated days of enrollment (National PACE Association, 1996b). Table 5.2 summarizes site-specific data for inpatient utilization. These numbers are significantly less than what would be expected for a nursing home certified group of adults over

TABLE 5.1 PACE Covered Services

1. The PACE service package includes, but is not limited to, all current Medicare and Medicaid services. All usual limitations and conditions for covered services are waived.
2. The PACE provider must provide its participants with access to medical care and other services, applicable 24 hours per day, 7 days a week, 365 days per year.
3. At a minimum each PACE provider shall provide the following services:
   a. Multidisciplinary assessment and treatment planning;
   b. Primary care services including physician and nursing services;
   c. Social work services;
   d. Restorative therapies, including physical therapy, occupational therapy and speech therapy;
   e. Personal care and supportive services;
   f. Nutritional counseling;
   g. Recreational therapy;
   h. Transportation;
   i. Meals;
   j. Medical specialty services including, but not limited to: anesthesiology, audiology, cardiology, dentistry, dermatology, gastroenterology, gynecology, internal medicine, nephrology, neurosurgery, oncology, ophthalmology, oral surgery, orthopedic surgery, otorhinolaryngology, plastic surgery, pharmacy consulting services, podiatry, psychiatry, pulmonary disease, radiology, rheumatology, surgery, thoracic and vascular surgery, urology;
   k. Laboratory tests, x-rays and other diagnostic procedures;
   l. Drugs and biologicals;
   m. Prosthetics and durable medical equipment, corrective vision devices such as eyeglasses and lenses, hearing aids, dentures, and repairs and maintenance for these items;
   n. Acute inpatient care:
      i. ambulance;
      ii. emergency room care and treatment room services;
      iii. semi-private room and board;
      iv. general medical and nursing services;
      v. medical surgical/intensive care/coronary care unit, as necessary;
      vi. laboratory tests, x-rays and other diagnostic procedures;
      vi. drugs and biologicals;
      viii. blood and blood derivatives;
      ix. surgical care, including the use of anesthesia;
      x. use of oxygen;
      xi. physical, speech, occupational, and respiratory therapies; and
      xii. social services.
   o. Nursing facility care:
      i. semi-private room and board;
      ii. physician and skilled nursing services;
      iii. custodial care;
      iv. personal care and assistance;
      v. drugs and biologicals;
      vi. physical, speech, occupational, and recreational therapies, if necessary;
      vii. social services; and
      viii. medical supplies and appliances.
   p. Additional services determined necessary by the multidisciplinary team.
4. Emergency Care
5. Urgent Care

Note. From *PACE Protocol, 1995.* OnLok, Inc., San Francisco, CA.

TABLE 5.2 PACE Cross-Site Comparison Inpatient Utilization 1992–1995

Location Entered	SF	E. Boston	Portland	Columbia	Milwaukee	Denver	Bronx	Rochester	Sacramento	El Paso	Oakland
Capitation	11/83	6/90	6/90	10/90	11/90	10/91	2/92	5/92	5/94	6/94	4/95
HOSPITAL DAYS/1000/ANNUM:											
1992	1320	3240	1800	2520	5520	4920	4800	5280	4320	6840	2280
1993	1800	2760	1680	960	2760	4440	7920	3240	3360	6000	4080
1994	1080	4320	1080	1200	3480	2520	4440	3720	2760	3000	3360
1995	1200	2760	1440	480	3000	2880	5040	3000	1800	2280	2040
AVERAGE LENGTH OF STAY IN HOSPITAL:											
1992	4.8	8.0	4.4	3.5	10.6	5.5	9.3	9.5	8.6	8.9	6.3
1993	5.2	3.8	3.2	2.9	5.5	5.0	12.9	7.7	7.6	9.0	9.2
1994	4.1	6.5	2.1	2.8	6.1	4.6	9.1	6.7	6.2	6.8	5.2
1995	4.1	5.4	2.7	1.9	5.9	4.5	5.2	6.9	6.3	4.4	4.1

Note. From National PACE Association (1996b). *A PACE profile 1996.* Brochure. San Francisco, CA: Author.

age 80. Freedom from the eligibility restraints of the fee-for-service system of reimbursements allows the PACE providers to create comprehensive care plans that truly reflect the needs of the frail participants and implement them in an integrated system of health-care services.

Integrated Care Through the Interdisciplinary Team

The interdisciplinary team is the central mechanism through which care is planned and provided. This interdisciplinary team model of care management reflects the biopsychosocial philosophy of the PACE model and recognizes that the day center and home health workers and van drivers have a perspective to offer in care planning and implementation that is equal in importance to that of the more traditional nurse and physician providers. The coordination of care and integration of acute- and long-term care services that characterize the PACE model are developed through constant attention to effective group process within each PACE site's interdisciplinary team (Eleazer, Baskins, Egbert, Johnson, & Wilson, 1994).

Each participant receives a thorough evaluation by a physician, nurse, social worker, nutritionist, activity/recreation therapist, and rehabilitation specialist. At several sites, pharmacists, optometrists, audiologists, dentists, and podiatrists are also included in the core interdisciplinary team. Evaluations and interdisciplinary team conferences are completed at intake and then quarterly to determine the needs of each participant and to establish the individualized comprehensive care plan. Unscheduled assessments and team meetings are performed whenever there is a major change in a participant's status or plan of care. The core interdisciplinary team is responsible for planning and coordinating care across all sites of care: home, the adult day health care center (referred to as the PACE Center), acute hospital, and, if necessary, the nursing home.

Participants and caregivers are involved in all phases of this evaluation and care plan process. Because the PACE model operates outside of the traditional Medicare/Medicaid entitlement-based allotment of services, there is maximum flexibility for the interdisciplinary team to negotiate details of the plan of care with the participants and caregivers and optimize the match between participants' needs and the services provided.

Implementation of treatment plans by the primary-care providers (PCPs), who also formulate them and monitor results of treatment, is an important characteristic of the PACE model. Services are allocated and rendered efficiently based on the needs assessment; outcomes of treatment become apparent to the care providers; and adjustments can be made quickly. The inclusion of the primary-care physician as an active team member who is present at team meetings is unique to the PACE model and insures that the medical and psychosocial issues are dealt with in a truly integrated fashion.

Ongoing Team Functions

A case example may help illustrate how the interdisciplinary team cares for participants in this model, both on an ongoing basis and during acute illness.

Ms. M is a 79-year-old Black female with multiple medical problems including the following:

- Severe emphysema
- Schizoaffective disorder
- Depression
- Gastroesophageal reflux disease
- Osteoarthritis
- Obesity
- Diabetes mellitus
- Parkinson's Disease

On enrollment in PACE, Ms. M needed assistance with dressing and bathing and supervision when transferring and walking. She had bladder incontinence approximately 2 times per week and occasional bowel incontinence. She required multiple medications.

Primary Care

Ms. M is managed by a nurse practitioner and primary-care internist who monitor her multiple medical problems. They work closely with other members of the team to optimize medical management. Ms. M is seen by the physician at least quarterly for reevaluation and is seen by her nurse practitioner 3 or 4 times during the month. Either the nurse practitioner or the physician may see her for episodic problems. Exacerbations of her emphysema occur several times each month and require close monitoring.

Nursing

Nursing responsibilities involve following the patient in the PACE Center 5 days per week. Nursing checks laboratory results including blood glucoses. Nursing also monitors vital signs at least twice a week, monitors medication compliance, administers nebulizer treatments, and monitors for episodic problems including exacerbations of Ms. M's emphysema and mental illness. Nurses communicate frequently with the family about any intercurrent problems and have worked with family members to improve bowel and bladder continence.

Home Care

Personal care aide and homemaker services provided through home care include assistance with bathing, mouth care, nail care, skin care, dressing, and toileting as well as housekeeping chores including cleaning the bathroom and kitchen, periodically assisting with meal preparation, doing laundry, and shopping. Home care provides medication reminders when Ms. M's primary caregiver is not available. Home care assists with nebulizer treatments at home and trains the caregiver to give nebulizer treatments and monitor home oxygen. Further, home care makes home assessments to assure that the home is accessible; that security is maintained; that plumbing, electricity, heating/air conditioning, refrigerator, and stove are all in working order; that there is access to laundry facilities; and that a smoke detector is present and functioning.

Pharmacy

The pharmacist is very active in this case by assisting with patient compliance through the use of Medisets and therapeutic drug monitoring. When the patient initially arrived in the program, she had significant polypharmacy and was taking ten prescribed medications, two over-the-counter medications, and two homeopathic remedies. The pharmacists worked closely with the physician to reduce the number of prescribed medications from ten to five. The pharmacist also monitors renal function and allergies and watches for drug interactions and adverse drug reactions.

Social Work

The social worker has been responsible for evaluating the informal support network at least quarterly, following up on caregiver status, and checking for caregiver burnout. The social worker works closely with the other members of the team in this case to assure that the patient's needs are being met. She has assisted with family counseling as needed. Family counseling and caregiver support have been particularly important in view of the number of Ms. M's psychiatric problems.

Rehabilitation

Physical therapy has worked closely with Ms. M to assist her in maintaining her ability to walk. Ms. M is at significant risk of losing her ability to walk because of the combination of osteoarthritis, hypoxia, and complications of her steroid therapy. The physical therapist provides maintenance physical therapy to help her maintain her ability to walk for short distances. The patient participates in an exercise group. Home assessment by the physical therapist identified the need for a tub grab bar to improve home safety.

Occupational therapy identified a reduction in the range of motion of both shoulders secondary to adhesive capsulitis. Active and passive range of motion has improved this condition and hopefully will prevent further deterioration.

Nutritional Services

Ms. M has diabetes mellitus, which is worse when she takes Prednisone for her obstructive lung disease. She follows a diet low in concentrated sweets, and her dietician helps to monitor her weight, serum albumin, and glucose. Ms. M has been well controlled off all medications. Previously she intermittently required insulin or oral hypoglycemic agents to control her blood sugar.

Recreational Therapy

Recreational therapy is involved with the patient in large group activities as well as arts, crafts, exercise group, and music therapy. The patient has an interest in scripture study and religious activities and participates in religious activities twice a week at the day health center.

Transportation

Transportation helps to monitor the patient's home situation on a daily basis during the week. Any problems identified at home or in conversations with the patient are relayed to nursing, social work, the PCP or nurse practitioner.

The above case example reflects the interdisciplinary nature of Ms. M's care. The actual providers of service sit on the interdisciplinary team meeting to plan her care. Areas of critical importance are monitored by multiple disciplines, a necessary redundancy that has helped to reduce the frequency and severity of her episodic illnesses.

Team Management of an Acute Medical Problem

Frail elderly people with multiple medical problems often have exacerbations of medical or social situations that may result in acute hospitalization.

The ability of the interdisciplinary team to manage these cases is a tremendous asset to the program. In the example of Ms. M her medical problems frequently exacerbate her emphysema. One illustration of how such an exacerbation can be managed by a team of people may be useful.

On December 4, 1995, Ms. M developed increasing shortness of breath, and her caregiver informed transportation and nursing at the center that she was not walking well. The patient was transported to the PACE Center, where further evaluation took place. Nursing was responsible for initial physical assessment and vital signs, which revealed a temperature of 101.2°. The physician was notified and Ms. M's assessment revealed that she had pneumonia. The physician contacted the family to reconfirm Ms. M's advance health-care directives. These included conservative care with no cardiopulmonary resuscitation and avoidance of hospitalization where possible. The physician, nurse practitioner, and home care professionals discussed the acute situation and decided to manage the patient at home with close monitoring and follow-up in the PACE Center.

Ms. M had intravenous and blood work access placed; labs were drawn by nursing. She was started on IV steroids for her exacerbation of obstructive airway disease and antibiotics for her pneumonia. Her respiratory distress was worse, and nebulizer treatments were initiated. Nursing and home care confirmed her caregiver's ability to administer nebulizer treatment at home. Pharmacy was involved in assuring medication compliance. Home care provided increased monitoring and assistance at home with her daily living activities by increasing nursing and personal care aide time. The patient required a wheelchair, which was obtained through home care. By December 6, she was doing considerably better and was switched to oral medications. She continued to improve without requiring further intervention.

Team members involved in coordinating the care described above included staff from nursing services, home health nursing, home health personal care aides, physician services, nurse practitioner services, pharmacy services, and transportation. These support services supplemented the caregivers' activities at home to allow the patient to stay at home without requiring acute hospitalization.

Prior to enrolling in PACE, the patient was cared for in a fee-for-service environment. In the year prior to enrollment, she required multiple hospitalizations related to exacerbations of emphysema or her mental illness. (These two problems seemed to exacerbate each other. For example, if Ms. M was hospitalized for emphysema, her mental condition would deteriorate, and vice versa). The fee-for-service environment did not allow the level of coordination to provide her care at home; nor did it allow for close monitoring to detect problems early so that they could be addressed and hospitalization could be prevented. Ms. M spent several weeks in a nursing home prior to enrolling in PACE since the fee-for-service system was not able to care for her at home.

PACE provided a number of benefits not available in traditional care. Transportation, coordinated care, monitoring of medical and mental problems at the PACE Center, and home care all helped prevent institutionalization. Ms. M's socialization improved and she was pleased with improvements in her quality of life. Her acute problems are now usually managed without hospitalization, reflecting her preferences and also lowering health-care costs.

There are a number of models of care that allow for multidisciplinary or interdisciplinary team care. However, the PACE model is unique in its combination of interdisciplinary care combined with the use of the PACE Center, its seamless coordination across the acute and long-term care systems, and its integrated financing. This seamless, integrated system of care is of great value in treating frail elders who want to remain in the community.

The importance of primary care in the model can not be overemphasized. A critical member of the interdisciplinary team is the PCP. The PCP is responsible for judicious use of the program's most expensive services: acute-care services. One of the challenges faced by the PACE sites is to successfully recruit and retain physicians who are both well qualified and experienced in dealing with frail elderly people and who also work well as members of true interdisciplinary teams in this nontraditional practice. The PCP must be able to respect the disciplines of the other team members as well as the members themselves. A working knowledge of the other disciplines may not be present on the PCP's first day on the job, but within a short period of time he or she must come to recognize the strengths and capabilities of other members of the team. Since a large portion of care will be rendered or managed through other team members, PCPs must be willing to share responsibility, recognizing that their other voice is just one of several, and trust the team members to provide for the participant.

While the PCP's judgement in medical decisions will be paramount, the team will have a significant say in psychosocial aspects that may override some medical decisions. For example, a patient may be medically capable of having a coronary artery bypass graft, but may have clearly expressed to the nurse and social worker on the team a wish not to have any life-prolonging surgery or hospitalizations. Such patients may be reluctant to tell their PCP of their decision for fear of somehow "disappointing the doctor." The PCP in the PACE project must be open to the opinions and recommendations of other members of the team in such situations, including those of the nurse's aides and drivers. To help identify this particular attribute, some sites conduct team interviews of physician applicants. This team interview process helps identify members who are unlikely to interact well with other team members.

One of the authors, GPE, a PACE medical director, recounts the following story:

> We were approximately 2 years into site development when our primary-care physician resigned. Our census growth had done reasonably well, and we were actually at a point at which we needed two primary-care physicians. We were considering several applicants. One applicant had previous experience with multidisciplinary teams working in a nursing home setting. This individual interviewed well, making definite eye contact with all members of the team. He responded well to questions and showed insight into the motivations behind questions. The second physician interviewed had no previous experience with interdisciplinary teams. However, her eye contact and interaction with all members of the team went well. She readily acknowledged her lack of knowledge of some of the disciplines and expressed an interest in learning more about how those disciplines helped provide care for this frail elderly population. She also indicated strong willingness to work as a "team player." The third physician interviewed responded differently. When questioned by members of the team, he directed his responses to the medical director only. This was evident by eye contact, body language, and spoken content. He showed poor insight into the value of other disciplines and did not appear to have any interest in working as a team player. Interestingly, this particular applicant had an excellent curriculum vitae and without the team interview would have been favorably considered for the position. The decision was to hire the first two physicians, who have remained with the program for 5 years. They have functioned very effectively as interdisciplinary team members.

Another characteristic felt to be predictive of physicians' success in this model is the ability to be flexible, yet diplomatically assertive. For example, physicians need to be flexible about the site of care delivery. Pneumonia may be treated at home, in the adult day health center, or in the hospital. Physicians who are more rigid are unlikely to succeed in PACE. One physician in the program was adamant that all patients with pneumonia required 7 days of IV antibiotics administered in the hospital setting. This physician was unable to adapt his practice style to the PACE model and left the program after only a few months. Physicians must be flexible in working with families and other members of the team. Discipline lines are often blurred in this model. Physicians who are rigid in their concept of discipline lines are often not happy in this model of integrated, interdisciplinary care. Several sites have reported unofficial "markers" that seem to be predictors of poor adaptation in this model. For example, physicians who refuse to do foot care, to discuss social issues with families, or to assist nursing staff and nursing aides in helping transfer patients in and out of beds and wheelchairs may be less likely to be successful in PACE. In short, an attitude of "That's not my job" or "That job is beneath me" is unlikely to lend itself to building the team approach to patient care.

Sites have hired a variety of physician specialists, including general internists, family physicians, and geriatricians. A 1992 survey by the PACE medical director of the 25 PCPs in PACE showed that 21 were internists and 4 were family medicine physicians; 80% were board-certified and 40% had certificates of added qualifications in geriatrics (C. Eng, personal communication, 1992). There are individual site variations depending on the availability and training of physicians in each location. Regardless of specialty, successful PCPs in PACE are generally willing to tackle difficult medical problems and complex medical cases without consulting multiple specialists. Physicians who are not comfortable with handling complicated, frail geriatric patients generally don't do well in the model. Further, it is important for sites to have PCPs who interact well with subspecialists and are respected by subspecialists, since subspecialty care often needs to be modified to fit in this model. The PCP at most, but not all, PACE sites continues to monitor and direct complicated care, including postoperative management and ICU care. Sites where the PCP remains "in control" of the patient tend to have a lower utilization of inpatient services and a lower number of acute care days.

Individual sites have reported different interactions between the PCPs and subspecialists ranging from close collaboration to confrontation. The South Carolina site and East Boston site illustrate some of these differences.

At the South Carolina site, the PCPs work closely with a small group of subspecialists, trying to use the same individual subspecialists within a group practice, if at all possible. The result is that many of these subspecialists are familiar with the program and have a high level of trust. This trust is based on a personal relationship and knowledge of the capabilities of the PACE PCPs and the support that the program itself provides. As a result, the PCPs have been able to effect rather dramatic changes in the practice patterns of these subspecialists. For example, surgical lengths of hospital stay for lower extremity amputation are often less than 1 day, with close follow-up by the PCP either in the nursing home, at the adult day health center, or at home. The consulting surgeons have been willing to accept this change after several years of familiarity with the staff physicians and the capabilities of this program. They understand that patients will receive extremely close monitoring and that any complications will be promptly identified and brought to a surgeon's attention.

In East Boston, this experience has been different. The Boston area has one of the highest rates of hospital utilization and also one of the highest per capita subspecialist-to-patient ratios in the United States. There has been resistance on the part of the subspecialists in the community to PCP-directed patient care. The "community standard" has been early and frequent subspecialty care. Frequently, multiple subspecialists care for one frail elderly person with multiple medical problems. Patients and families have come to expect subspecialty care. The PCPs at this site have experienced particular difficulty in maintaining control of the case of a participant who requires hospitalization. Hospitalization often leads to subspecialist involvement. The medical community in East Boston is large, and consulting subspecialists often don't know or have personal relationships with the PCP, and are not familiar with the PACE program. PCPs in East Boston report difficulty in obtaining early discharge, but the services available there are unlike those available at the South Carolina site. Subspecialists have generally resisted modifying their practice patterns. Nevertheless, the East Boston site has continued to do well, which is a reflection of the PACE physicians' persistence in pursuing the model.

Flexibility

Not only is flexibility important on the part of physicians, but it also pertains to the way care is delivered. Complicated medical problems can be taken care of in a variety of health-care settings, including the nursing home, the PACE adult day care center, transitional housing, and the home of the patient. In addition, programs have the flexibility to provide unusual services that are not covered in traditional health-care systems. Sites often report that much of their pleasure in caring for patients is their ability to do "what makes sense." Often "what makes sense" could not be provided in the fee-for-service or other managed health plans. A few examples may help to illustrate this point.

A common problem among programs that serve indigent populations is substance abuse in caregivers. This results in danger to the elderly. Dealing with the combination of substance abuse and caregiving to a frail elder is difficult. This situation is often complicated when an elderly person lives in an area that is not served by public transportation and that suffers a high crime rate. Crime may have reached the point that even private taxi services will no longer go into a patient's neighborhood.

A participant living in this complicated situation is often best cared for by the PACE interdisciplinary team. Transportation is provided, and the team has the opportunity to monitor the situation closely and remove the elder should the situation deteriorate further. The team also has the ability to look for other housing arrangements in a safer area. Should the caregiver begin or increase substance abuse, the interdisciplinary team is likely to be aware of this and address the issue. In such situations, caregivers often spend the little household money available on alcohol or other drugs. This may result in the threat of eviction or turning off utilities. The interdisciplinary team has the ability to intervene and even pay the rent or the electric bill while trying either to arrange for a different caregiver or to get the caregiver into a treatment program. Most traditional health-care plans would have neither the resources to monitor the situation this closely, nor the flexibility to make temporary payments to prevent the elder from being evicted. In many traditional systems, such a situation would result in the elderly person's being admitted to the hospital for "social reasons" at a much higher cost to society. Alternatively, the electricity or gas would be turned off, which could potentially result in hypothermia, pneumonia, and other medical complications, also resulting in a preventable hospitalization.

The program's flexibility has raised the interest of the public and resulted in positive publicity for the model. A case cited in the *New York Times* in 1994 is illustrative (Tamar, 1994). In this case, a patient with hypertension, diabetes, peripheral vascular disease resulting in bilateral leg amputations, and blindness was managed by the program in a very effective way so that she could maintain her independence. The program assisted her in locating a safer housing situation and provided close monitoring and care of her medical problems. It even paid for deflea-ing her dog, since flea bites were felt to be a significant risk for her health, given her diabetes mellitus.

Integrated Financing

The PACE model can provide the entire spectrum of prevention, rehabilitation, acute care and long-term care services in the community setting because of Medicare and Medicaid waivers granted to PACE provider organizations (Shen & Iverson, 1992). These waivers free the provider organization from the normal benefit definitions and allow participant "lock-in," which suspends participants' freedom of choice of providers while they are enrolled in a PACE program. Each PACE site receives monthly capitation payments from Medicare, Medicaid, and, for individuals not eligible for Medicaid, private pay. Medicare bases its payment on the adjusted average per capital cost (AAPCC) methodology used to reimburse HMOs with Medicare risk plans. For PACE, the AAPCC is multiplied by a single frailty-adjustment factor. In 1995, the monthly Medicare capitation ranged from $737 to $1,623 across the PACE sites. The variation reflects different geographic rates of reimbursement by Medicare in the fee-for-service system. The Medicaid portion is negotiated state by state, with each state basing its reimbursement on what it pays for a comparable frail long-term care population (either home- and community-based or in a nursing home). Medicaid monthly capitation in 1995 ranged from $1,486 to $4,465, which is estimated to be 5% to 15% less than its costs for a similar population. Individuals ineligible for Medicaid pay the Medicaid portion of the capitated rate privately.

These funds are pooled by a PACE site and are used to provide participants with the services they need to maintain optimal health and function in the community. The PACE sites are financially at risk for the services provided. Because it cannot shift costs, the PACE model manages financial risk by keeping participants as healthy as possible through aggressive preventive health practices and frequent monitoring of their status in the clinics and day health centers (Kunz, 1996). This integrated system of financing provides the incentives for a win-win outcome. The healthier and more functional participants remain, the less likely it is that they will need to utilize the most expensive resources: acute care in the hospital and long-term care in the nursing home. As a result, participants and their caregivers will be more satisfied, and the PACE will be financially viable.

CURRENT STATUS OF THE PACE MODEL

As of December 1995, the 10 initial PACE sites operating under dual (Medicare and Medicaid) waivers were providing services to 2,709 clients eligible for placement in nursing homes. Because all enrollees in the PACE model must be certified for nursing home placement, multiple medical conditions and functional impairments are the norm (Table 5.3). In 1995, the average number of medical conditions for enrollees was 7.93, and the average number of dependencies in the activities of daily living (ADLs) for which enrollees received assistance was 2.65. Almost 100% are dependent in all instrumental activities of daily living (IADLs). Sixty percent had some type of cognitive impairment.

Demographic characteristics of current enrollees of the PACE models indicate that the targeting process is serving the intended frail nursing-home-eligible client. Demographics show an average age of 80 years, a predominance of the female sex, and a distribution of race or ethnicity that reflects the community or defined geographic area in which the PACE site is located. Among the 19 total sites at various stages of development

TABLE 5.3 1995 Cross-Site PACE Portrait Dual-Capitated Sites

Location CENSUS AS OF 12/31/95	SF	E. Boston	Portland	Columbia	Milwaukee	Denver	Bronx	Rochester	Sacramento	El Paso	Oakland	Average for Dual-Capitated Sites
	428	208	264	229	274	203	330	258	145	253	117	
Average No. Medical Conditions	7.00	8.50	8.30	6.40	9.00	7.40	7.20	9.50	4.90	11.00	6.80	7.93
Average ADL Dependencies	2.40	2.30	2.50	3.60	2.70	2.60	2.00	3.10	3.10	2.60	3.10	2.65
% of enrollees needing help with:												
Bathing	81%	89%	81%	93%	84%	85%	71%	88%	89%	76%	88%	83%
Dressing	63%	58%	63%	88%	66%	60%	59%	79%	74%	65%	74%	67%
Grooming	68%	84%	64%	90%	73%	76%	57%	86%	91%	60%	88%	74%
Toileting	48%	33%	49%	75%	55%	46%	35%	55%	59%	48%	46%	49%
Transfer	44%	24%	41%	54%	43%	39%	34%	52%	58%	53%	44%	44%
Walking	47%	22%	41%	55%	44%	42%	48%	47%	67%	68%	50%	48%
Feeding	18%	24%	34%	52%	40%	26%	16%	35%	23%	17%	58%	29%

*Capitated enrollees only; most service figures equal average number of services/enrollee/month.
Note. From National PACE Association (1996b). A PACE profile 1996. Brochure. San Francisco, CA: Author.

operating in 1995, 10 had a predominance of enrollees from one ethnic group, while nine sites had a mixture of three or more ethnicities represented. Forty-six percent of the enrollees are Caucasian, 24% are African American, 15% are Hispanic American, 14% are Asian, and 1% are "Other" (National PACE Association, 1996b).

The PACE project has demonstrated that the OnLok model of care can be successfully replicated in a variety of geographic areas and ethnic groups (Branch et al., 1995).

QUALITY IN THE PACE MODEL

From the beginnings of OnLok in the 1970s and continuing with the PACE model in the 1980s and 1990s, the systematic collection of patient data for the purpose of demonstrating the quality of life and care of its participants has been a major focus of provider organizations and their state and federal insurers. This section describes the evolution of quality assurance activities undertaken to date (Kipnis, 1996).

PACE is a demonstration project, and thus quality control activities are important to assure that the individual PACE sites are accurately replicating the OnLok model. Data collection has been handled through a program called DataPACE. Operational guidelines and the PACE protocol were developed to assure accurate replication.

DataPACE

Prior to the replication of the PACE model nationally, OnLok collected and used participant and service utilization data for management and evaluation purposes. This data set was refined for the PACE replication to include other variables to be used in the evaluation of the PACE project. Participant-specific intake, assessment, and service utilization data is collected and coded according to the guidelines in the *PACE Data Collection Manual*. The definition of data and the manner in which it is collected may be changed to meet changes in Health Care Financing Administration (HCFA) and state Medicaid agency reporting requirements and in response to requests from PACE providers. Any changes made in the data collection incorporate sufficient lead time to minimize transition difficulty. In this way, data uniformity is maintained across all PACE providers.

From this data, reports are generated quarterly and submitted to HCFA and state Medicaid agencies. The following statistical reports are included: Program Status Report, Sociodemographic Characteristics of Participants,

Health and Functional Status of Participants, and Service Utilization Summary. This uniform PACE Minimum Data Set allows the program to do cross-site comparisons and analyze trends over time on participants' health status and service utilization. This data set, called DataPACE, has allowed the PACE providers to assess whether or not they are achieving the goals of the program: serving the frail elderly, offering comprehensive services, and minimizing the use of acute hospitals and long-term care. The low disenrollment rates, as monitored by DataPACE, suggest a high degree of participant and caregiver satisfaction with the PACE model.

Operational Guidelines

The Operational Guidelines evolved from efforts by OnLok to implement and document its own standards of care, which focused on each discipline as well as on interdisciplinary functions. They incorporated community review of services provided through the medical advisory, utilization review, and ethics committees (Zawadski & Eng, 1988). Community review was felt to be important because of the population being served. These standards of care were incorporated in a test survey instrument for a multiagency team representing the state agencies involved in licensing and certification of the OnLok programs. The intent was to consolidate the multiple survey processes for the adult day health program, the clinic, the home health agency, and medical review surveys into one review that would reflect the integration of acute and long-term services being provided. These standards were disseminated to the PACE sites in 1989 as Operational Guidelines.

PACE Protocol

The PACE Protocol was developed as a cooperative effort in 1990 by OnLok, HCFA, states participating in PACE replication and, importantly, the PACE sites themselves to establish the basic standards of care for PACE providers and to assure accurate replication of the OnLok model of care. The Protocol originally served as the specific legal instrument for implementing the PACE demonstration at the first 10 sites and provided the regulatory framework for core operating procedures and processes in the absence of formal federal and state regulation. In December 1993 the Protocol was updated to incorporate the experience of PACE providers in implementing the model. Again, comments were received from HCFA and state Medicaid agency representatives, and the document has been finalized as of April 1995. It is intended to serve as the basic standard for PACE providers, except as it may be subsequently modified by law or regulation. Included in these standards are clear requirements for continuing the internal quality assurance activities *and* a plan for developing periodic on-site surveys to provide external oversight of the quality of care.

Preliminary Evaluation Studies of the PACE Model

A number of preliminary studies have looked at various aspects of the PACE program. Through contracts with the University of Minnesota Health Policy Center, HCFA has supported the Qualitative Analysis of the Program of All Inclusive Care for the Elderly (Kane, Illson, & Miller, 1992). HCFA also contracted with Abt Associates to provide an independent evaluation of the project. A preliminary report of the evaluation has been published (Branch et al., 1995). Additionally, in 1994, two independent studies of individual sites were completed: the "Palmetto SeniorCare Client Satisfaction Survey" by the South Carolina State Health and Human Services Finance Commission, Columbia, SC (South Carolina State Health and Human Services Finance Commission, 1994) and "Independent Living for Seniors: A 3-year Assessment of Perceptions and Impact of Program" by the Center for Governmental Research, Inc., Rochester, NY (Pryor, 1994).

Kane's qualitative analysis of the experience of the first PACE replication sites during the start-up phase of 1990-91 identified slower than anticipated enrollment, partially a result of the reluctance of enrollees to change physicians and resistance to adult day health care. Branch's evaluation of 1993 program status demonstrated a continuation of these issues, but found that the PACE sites were already responding by becoming more flexible in their care plans and relaxing day care attendance requirements (Branch, 1995). Branch's study raised the issue of whether the PACE program was preferentially taking less frail clients than intended. HCFA found no evidence to support this charge (Clauser et al., 1996). Table 5.3 provides a portrait of PACE participants, including dependencies in ADLs.

The South Carolina State Health and Human Services Finance Commission conducted a survey of Palmetto SeniorCare participants and their caregivers and found a high degree of satisfaction with the services offered by this PACE site. Seventy-four percent of respondents felt their medical care was "excellent" or "very good." Most (63%) felt the medical care was an improvement over their previous source of care, and the majority of both participants and their caregivers felt that the quality of their life had improved because of the program. This type of satisfaction survey also helps the PACE sites identify specific problems that they can address in ongoing quality improvement; for example, irregular van pick-up and drop-off, participant and caregiver participation in decision-making, and more accessible support groups.

The 3-year evaluation of the Rochester PACE site by the Center of Governmental Research examined whether the program could market itself effectively and attract sufficient enrollees, would be perceived as improving the quality of life of the participants, and could effectively reduce the utilization of acute hospital care. This study demonstrated that the Rochester PACE site was successful in each of these three domains. The low disenrollment rate (3–5%) also suggests high client satisfaction (Kunz & Shannon, 1996).

Review by the Community Health Accreditation Program (CHAP)

In 1993, the Community Health Accreditation Program (CHAP) served as an independent third party to assess the quality of care at five PACE sites. Building on the Operational Guidelines and the PACE Protocol, CHAP and OnLok collaboratively developed a consolidated survey instrument that addressed both administrative and clinical activities. This instrument was then applied by an interdisciplinary survey team that consisted of a physician, nurse, social worker, and peer reviewer from a PACE site that was operating under full risk. One of the authors, Marsha Fretwell, served as a physician site surveyor for this effort. Two-day on-site surveys culminated in a final interactive meeting where issues were discussed and remedies proposed. Exceptional quality and coordination of care were demonstrated at all five sites. Recommendations for improvement focused on continuing attention to the development of truly integrated team meetings and care management and improved methods for documenting the high quality of patient outcomes.

Development of a Quality Assurance System for PACE

In March 1996, Robert Kane and some of his colleagues from the University of Minnesota School of Public Health completed a project that developed a quality assurance system for the PACE program (Kane, 1996). Funded through HCFA, this project evaluated (1) the ability of structured implicit review of participant charts to demonstrate differences in the quality of care; (2) the inter-rater reliability of reviewers using this type of chart review; and (3) the utility of reviewers from different professional backgrounds. Structured implicit review is a type of chart review that depends on clinician reviewers to use their clinical judgment rather than explicit criteria to assess the quality of care. The structured approach to implicit review uses trained reviewers, specific questions to focus the reviewers' attention, and direct reference to sites of relevant data in the medical records. The results of this project were mixed. On one hand, this approach to quality assessment did detect differences in patterns of care among sites. (The ratings of the overall quality care management showed 5% as poor or worse and 22% as very good.) On the other hand, the chart review process was very time-consuming, and did not enhance inter-rater reliability. Finally, nurse practitioners performed more consistently than physicians.

This project demonstrates the challenge of defining and assessing quality of care for this group of frail older adults who routinely have multiple interacting medical and functional problems. Because OnLok and the PACE models represent a truly innovative effort to integrate all dimensions of care for their frail participants, there are no preexisting models for effectively comparing the quality of care that these programs offer.

NATIONAL PACE ASSOCIATION

The National PACE Association (NPA) has received funding from the Robert Wood Johnson Foundation to develop a national accreditation program for the PACE providers (Kipnis, 1996). The National PACE Association was formed in June 1994 to increase the provision of higher quality, comprehensive health-care services to frail older adults in the United States through PACE. The NPA sponsors educational events and leads the PACE sites' efforts in information dissemination, advocacy, and quality assurance. The NPA's board of directors consists of representatives from sites in full financial risk. In the area of quality assurance, the objectives of the NPA are to create model standards and performance measures with, and for, the PACE providers and to establish a national accreditation process for the PACE sites.

The NPA has initiated a work group consisting of NPA staff, experienced sites' program and administrative staff, and a National Accreditation Advisory Committee to provide ongoing feedback to the work group (Kipnis, 1996). These groups will refine and augment existing structural and process elements from the PACE Protocol and standards developed collaboratively with CHAP and also identify outcome standards. Structural standards will cover organizational capacity, staffing, and financial risk reserve requirements. Process standards will include the interdisciplinary team process, responsiveness in addressing changes in participant condition, and participant involvement in treatment planning. Proposed outcome standards will include participant and family satisfaction, disenrollment rate, mortality rate, and changes in functional status.

Established accrediting bodies are either facility-based or tied to a specific type of service and therefore do not fully serve the NPA's need. The NPA will build on the knowledge of existing experts to develop an accreditation process that addresses the unique requirements of the PACE providers.

COST AND REIMBURSEMENT

The PACE program is designed to integrate service delivery and all financing for acute and long-term care. Funding is derived predominantly from Medicare and Medicaid, although at some sites participants pay part the Medicaid portion out of pocket. In a few cases, participants pay all of the Medicaid portion, but many of these private pay clients are in a "spend down" program through which they will expand their existing resources to qualify for Medicaid. The two funding streams are combined so that for one monthly capitated rate all health-care services are provided to the participant.

Medicare rates for the PACE program are based on the average adjusted per capita cost (AAPCC) multiplied by a frailty adjuster. The AAPCC is determined by HCFA and represents the average per capita cost to Medicare for beneficiaries in a given county. The AAPCC includes the entire Medicare eligible population, which is predominantly healthy. Since PACE serves exclusively frail elderly who consume considerably more resources than the healthy, an adjustment for frailty is made to the rate. Studies by Gruenberg and his colleagues found that Medicare beneficiaries requiring nursing home care cost between 2.63 and 3.6 times the AAPCC for the general Medicare population (Gruenberg, Tompkins, & Porell, 1990). In PACE, programs receive 95% of the AAPCC for the beneficiaries in their community multiplied by a frailty factor of 2.39. Further studies by Gruenberg and his colleagues suggest that PACE yields Medicare savings of at least 14% and possibly as much as 39% (Gruenberg, Rumshiskaya, & Kaganova, 1993).

Medicaid funding for PACE varies from state to state. Medicaid rates are negotiated between each site and its respective Medicaid agency in its state. There is no preestablished formula, although all states evaluate their PACE rate against their expenditures for comparably frail (that is, nursing-home certified) individuals who are receiving long-term care services outside of PACE. The difficulty in setting rates for Medicaid has been to determine to which population and which level of care the PACE rate should be linked. In general, most states have limited Medicaid capitation payments to PACE to a percentage of the negotiated base rates that they calculated for a similar population. Rates are set at a fraction of the state's expenditures for a similar long-term care population. Table 5.4 summarizes the capitated payments for Medicare/Medicaid and PACE in 1996. Total monthly capitation by site varied from a low $2,530 in Denver to a high of $5,760 in the Bronx, reflecting considerable differences in fee-for-service spending across states.

Limitations of the Model

The original purpose of the PACE demonstration project was to determine whether the OnLok model of care could be replicated in other geographic

TABLE 5.4 PACE Capitation Rates 1996

PACE Site State—City	Medicare Rate	Medicaid Rate	Total Rate
CA—San Francisco	1,227	2,213	3,440
CA—Sacramento	1,137	1,865	3,002
CA—Oakland	1,249	2,245	3,494
CO—Denver	1,044	1,486	2,530
MA—Boston	1,433	2,103	3,536
NY—Bronx	1,754	4,006	5,760
NY—Rochester	989	2,928	3,917
OR—Portland	920	1,704	2,624
SC—Columbia	813	2,144	2,957
TX—El Paso	966	1,819	2,785
WI—Wisconsin	1,014	2,137	3,151
Pace Median	Medicare 1,044	Medicaid 2,137	Total 3,151

Notes:
Plus Share of Cost collected by OnLok (CA), Co, TX.
Co—Medicare rate shown is average paid in 3 counties.
NY–Bronx—Medicaid rate is a weighted average of SNF rate of $4,124 and ICF rate of $2,550.
SC—Medicaid rate is net after adjustment to revenue.

areas and in other ethnic populations. OnLok developed in a relatively small area of San Francisco serving the Chinatown and North Beach areas. The population was predominately ethnic Chinese. The results of the PACE demonstration so far have shown that the model's effectiveness is not limited to high-density urban areas or ethnic Chinese (Branch et al., 1995; Kane, Illson, & Miller, 1992). The sites selected to replicate the model have been geographically dispersed, although most sites are in urban areas and a true rural version of the model has yet to be tested. Transportation can be a limiting factor in the program's ability to bring participants into the adult day health center. In more rural areas, transportation is likely to be an even greater problem.

The OnLok model is based in part on attendance at the PACE center, a facility that offers services typically available in a primary-care clinic, adult day health care center, and rehabilitation facility. One of the reasons participants have given for not enrolling in a PACE program is the expectation that they attend the center (Kane et al., 1992). It is unclear whether less frequent center attendance would still allow the programs to provide adequate and cost-effective services to elders. Some sites are experimenting with reducing the amount of center attendance required for participants who prefer to remain at home.

The census growth of the PACE sites has been slower than would have been predicted (Branch et al., 1995; Kane et al., 1992). Besides the requirement related to center attendance, another commonly cited reason that participants do not enroll is that they do not want to switch the PCP (Kane et al., 1992). Limited census growth has a financial impact on the sites, thus hampering expansion and increasing risks.

A further limitation of the program has been that it serves mainly the dually eligible (Medicare plus Medicaid) population. A minority of elders nationwide qualify for Medicaid, and the applicability of this program to nonindigent populations remains to be seen.

Although there is considerable enthusiasm for the PACE model of care, it is important to recognize that it has been designed for a small, targeted group of frail elderly. Clauser et al. (1996) have pointed out that only a small subset of the nursing home eligible population is appropriate for this model. Not only must potential clients meet state-determined nursing home eligibility requirements, but they and/or their support network must want to prevent institutionalization. In keeping with its philosophy, PACE makes a deliberate attempt to prevent institutionalization and acute hospitalization (Kane, 1995). Many elders (or their caregivers) may not support this philosophy of care and thus would not be appropriate for this model.

Future Directions

As has been noted, with the success of the replication of the OnLok model of care, the PACE projects have formed the National PACE Association (NPA). The interest in this model has grown tremendously, with nearly fifty organizations all developing PACE programs or exploring the feasibility of developing them. The Balanced Budget Act of 1997 designated provider status for PACE. At the time of this writing, the Health Care Financing Administration is in the process of developing the necessary regulations. The NPA, recognizing the importance of quality standards for long-term viability of the model, has received a grant from the Robert Wood Johnson Foundation to develop accreditation standards for the PACE model, as has also been previously noted above.

Several sites have received grants to explore replicating the PACE model in other populations. The South Carolina site is moving forward with a plan to apply this model of care to frail children (Brown, Byrd, & Baskins, 1995). Massachusetts is considering replicating the model for AIDS patients, while the Bronx site has applied the model successfully to younger disabled clients eligible for nursing home care with reduced use of institutional services. Hopefully, the model will be applicable to a number of special, frail populations.

CONCLUSIONS

The PACE demonstration project has shown that the interdisciplinary model of care developed at OnLok for frail elders can be successfully replicated in diverse geographic areas and ethnic groups. The model is successful in reducing acute care hospitalization and nursing home placement. Client satisfaction has remained high. Although the final evaluation of the project is still pending, the project shows considerable promise.

REFERENCES

Ansak, M. L. (1990). The OnLok model: Consolidating care and financing. *Generations, LT Financing, 12,* 73–74.

Branch, L. G., Coulam, R. F., & Zimmerman, Y. A. (1995). The PACE Evaluation: Initial findings. *The Gerontologist, 35,* 349–359.

Brown, T. E., Byrd, M. D., & Baskins, J. P. (1995). Managed care for persons needing long-term care: Implications for home health. *Journal of Home Health Care Practice, 7*, 45–52.
CHAP Quality Association. (1993). *Program of All Inclusive Care for the Elderly: Summary of findings*. Available from CHAP, 350 Hudson St., New York, New York 10014.
Clauser, S. B., Kidder, D., & Mauser, K. (1996). "The PACE Evaluation." Letter to the editor. *Gerontologist, 36*, 7–8.
Eleazer, G. P. (1995). Integrating acute and long-term care: The PACE project. In J. C. Romeis, R. M. Coe, & J. E. Morley, *Applying health services research to long-term care* (pp. 208–217). New York: Springer Publishing Company.
Eleazer, G. P., Baskins, J. P., Egbert, J. R., Johnson, C. D., & Wilson, L. (1994). Managed care for the frail elderly: The PACE project. *Journal of the South Carolina Medical Association, 90*, 586–592.
Eng, C. (1987). Multidisciplinary approach to medical care: The OnLok model. *Clinical Report on Aging, 1*, 5–7.
Freidman, S. M., Barton, L. C., Rathous, P., Goldsborough, D., Elan, R. D., & Clark, M. (1995, April 25). *Risk factors for nursing home admission within PACE*. Paper presented at the 8th Annual PACE Forum.
Gruenberg, L., Leutz, W., & Silva, A. (1993). *An improved Medicare payment system for the social/HMO*. Unpublished Final Report to HCFA.
Gruenberg, L., Rumshiskaya, A., & Kaganova, J. (1993). *An analysis of expected Medicare costs for participants in the PACE demonstration*. Cambridge, MA: The Long Term Care Data Institute.
Gruenberg, L., Tompkins, C., & Porell, F. (1990). *Capitation rates for the frail elderly*. Bigel Institute Health Policy, Brandeis University. Baltimore, MD: United States Health Care Financing Administration.
Kane, R. L. (1995). Health care reform and the care of older adults. *Journal of the American Geriatrics Society, 43*, 702–706.
Kane, R. L. (1996). *A quality assurance system for the Program for All inclusive Care for the Elderly (PACE)*. Minneapolis, MN: Institute for Health Care Research.
Kane, R. L., Illson, L. H., & Miller, N. A. (1992). Qualitative analysis of the Program of All Inclusive Care for the Elderly (PACE). *Gerontologist, 32*, 771–780.
Kipnis, J. (1996). *Developing a national accreditation program for PACE*. Unpublished manuscript.
Kunz, E., & Shannon, K. (1996). PACE: Managed care for the frail elderly. *American Journal of Managed Care, 2*, 301–304.
National PACE Association. (1996b). *A PACE profile 1996*. Brochure. San Francisco: Author.
National PACE Association. (1996a). *1995 Cross-site comparisons PACE*. San Francisco: Author.
Operational Guidelines (revised. June 1993). *California Program of All-inclusive Care for the Elderly (PACE)/pre-PACE Operational Guidelines: Program flexibility*. Unpublished document. San Francisco: OnLok, Inc.

Pryor, D. E. (1994). Independent living for seniors: A 3-year assessment of perceptions and impact of program. Rochester, NY: Center for Governmental Research.

Shen, J., & Iverson, A. (1992). PACE: A capitated model towards long-term care. *Henry Ford Hospital Medical Journal, 40,* 41–44.

South Carolina State Health and Human Services Finance Commission. (1994). *Palmetto SeniorCare Client Satisfaction Survey.* Columbia, SC: South Carolina Department of Health and Human Services.

Tamar, L. (1994, February 14). Keeping elderly at home and care affordable. *New York Times,* p. 1.

Zawadski, R. T., & Eng, C. (1988). Case management in capitated long-term care. *Health Care Financing Administration Review* (Supp.), 75–81.

6
Implications of Managed Care for Older Persons

Robert Newcomer
Charlene Harrington
Robert L. Kane

The current emphasis on managed care by Medicare stems, at least in part, from the cost savings and programmatic care coordination efficiencies assumed to be associated with this form of service delivery. These assumptions form part of the $99.4 billion Medicare savings projected by the Balanced Budget Act of 1997. Less optimistic forecasters note that historically Medicare HMOs have tended to be more attractive to relatively healthy beneficiaries. As a consequence, managed health care for the elderly may proportionately underserve frail and high-risk cases in the population. Managed care practices of achieving cost savings through restrictions on the length of physician office visits, and controlled access to tests, procedures, and specialty care, may also underserve those in greater need. Such restrictions are thought to induce the less healthy to disenroll, gaining favorable financial advantages to the plans, while shifting high-cost patients to fee-for-service. Paralleling these concerns is the difficulty to date in structuring managed care systems that recruit members from persons dually eligible for Medicare and Medicaid.

To place these alternately hopeful and fearful scenarios into perspective, this chapter reviews the empirical literature related to effectiveness and quality of care within managed health care systems, and discusses approaches being developed within managed care plans for integrating care planning and delivery for persons considered at risk for disability or expensive care.

DEFINITION OF MANAGED HEALTH CARE

Managed care has many meanings within the field of aging and long-term care. For purposes of this discussion, we focus on health care and its interrelationship with the long-term care system. The most fundamental feature of managed health care is the "management" of physician practice. This occurs in the form of the selection and retention of physicians into eligible provider networks, utilization and practice pattern profiling and feedback, provider reimbursement, financial risk sharing or other financial incentives, physician organization, and practice guidelines. Varying combinations of these procedures are used within any one managed care plan or organization. As characterized by Miller and Luft (1994b), managed care plans include health maintenance organizations (HMOs), preferred provider organizations (PPOs),[1] and point of service (POS) plans.[2] Of these, HMOs have been most prevalent among elderly enrollees, and the subject of most of the evaluative literature.

HMOs come in a variety of forms. One is the prepaid group practice (or group model HMO) in which an administrative entity (e.g., Kaiser Health Plan) has an exclusive relationship with one or more large medical groups (e.g., the Permanente Medical Group). This contrasts with a network HMO (e.g., Pacificare Health Systems) where the medical group relationship is not exclusive. Staff model HMOs (e.g., Group Health Cooperative) are characterized by directly employing physicians. Finally, there is a mixed-model HMO (e.g., Health Plan of Nevada) in which the administrative intermediary may contract exclusively with medical groups and nonexclusively with solo practice physicians in the same area.

---

[1] Preferred provider organizations (i.e., PPOs) refer to the combination of financial intermediary organization and the network of providers with which it contracts to provide care. Providers in these organizations provide care to PPO enrollees on fee-for-service basis, usually at a discounted unit price from the community's "usual, customary, and reasonable" price. Often there may be a pre-set fee schedule. PPO enrollees come from employer groups, unions, and other groups with which the PPO has negotiated the opportunity to recruit such members. Providers (e.g., solo and group practice physicians, hospitals, mental health, and other providers) participating in a PPO usually have nonexclusive relationships with each other. Providers participate in PPOs to gain ready access to patients. The absence of risk sharing by providers in a PPO, places the incentives for utilization control on the PPO rather than the provider. PPO enrollment, historically, restricts coverage for primary care and some specialty services to the plan's network providers.

[2] Point of service plans (i.e., POS) are variations on the provider "lock-in" provisions of both HMO and PPO coverage. The distinguishing characteristic of a POS is that enrollees can be covered for services obtained outside of the HMO or PPO network providers. When this is done, service co-payments and deductibles are usually higher than they would be from a network provider. This type of coverage within an HMO is also called an "open-ended HMO plan." Both HMOs and PPOs are increasingly offering a point of service option for their enrollees.

ENROLLMENT AND PROVIDER PARTICIPATION

Managed care plans grew substantially during the 1980s as employers reacted to high rates of increase for indemnity health care insurance premiums. By 1995, nearly three-quarters of U.S. workers with health insurance received that coverage through some form of managed care. HMO plans covered 28% of employees, while PPOs and POSs covered 25% and 20%, respectively. Those covered by indemnity insurance had declined to 27%. These enrollments reflect almost a halving of those with indemnity coverage between 1993 and 1995 (Jenson, Morrisey, Gaffney, & Liston, 1997). The early movement from indemnity toward managed care coverage varied greatly by region of the country and local market area, but the trend toward capitation as the dominant payment method now seems established throughout the country. Some estimate that indemnity products will represent only about 10% of the insurance market by the turn of the century (Armstead, Elstein, & Gorman, 1995).

Managed care options have been available as a feature of Medicare since its inception in 1965, however, a shift to emphasize these arrangements occurred with the Tax Equity and Fiscal Responsibility Act (TEFRA) of 1982. This legislation authorized Medicare to implement full-risk HMOs and competitive medical plans. Under risk the contracted plan receives a prepayment for each enrollee and assumes financial risk for the actual costs of care. Prior to this, HMOs operated as fee-for-service providers for Medicare members, with reimbursement on the basis of billed service claims. Plans with risk contracts are often referred to as TEFRA HMOs or, more recently, as Medicare HMOs. The payment for each risk contract member is currently determined by a combination of their characteristics (i.e., age, gender, residence in a nursing home, Medicaid eligibility, reason for entitlement [e.g., aged vs. disabled]). The basis for these rates is the adjusted average per capita costs (AAPCC) determined for "rate cells" reflecting each of these characteristics. The AAPCC is calculated from Medicare reimbursed services under fee-for-service within the plan's catchment area. The Medicare capitation payment to managed care plans is 95% of the AAPCC for each member. The capitation payment methodology is intended to give managed care plans the incentives to control utilization, both by efficient use of resources and by preventive care.

The use of the AAPCC emphasizes the substantial variation in Medicare payments from place to place, a range of at least 100% (Kane & Friedman, 1997). The Balanced Budget Act has attempted to address these issues in several ways. Over time, the payment formula will move to a national rate instead of a local one. A minimum payment rate has been established. This rate offers a special boon to rural areas where the AAPCC has been especially low. Indeed, managed care organizations stand to make a substantial profit by enrolling residents under this new rate unless utilization increases dramatically.

Medicare beneficiary enrollment into a managed care plan is voluntary. Currently members can disenroll monthly, returning to fee-for-service or joining another managed care plan. This feature is also changing under Balanced Budget Act (BBA) provisions which permit only annual disenrollment, as is typical in group health plans. Annual lock-in may slow the growth in enrollments, but it facilitates care management and reduces the member's ability to leave a plan if benefit caps (such as annual drug coverage) are reached.

The incentives attracting risk contract enrollment are a reduction in out-of-pocket expenses for Medicare covered services and access to some benefits (such as prescription drugs) not otherwise covered by Medicare. Risk plan members are generally "locked" into the HMO's service provider network. However, as of 1996 some plans began to offer "point of service" options (i.e., access to non-network providers). This trend is expected to accelerate because of BBA provisions that encourage Medicare Choice plans. These feature point-of-service arrangements.

Basic Medicare benefits include: hospital, physician, limited skilled nursing facility use, skilled home health, and durable medical equipment. Federally qualified HMOs (and other managed care products) must provide these basic benefits, and cover all Medicare deductibles and coinsurance. Some plans charge co-payments and premiums, while others are offered at zero premium. Under the Medicare risk contract arrangement, managed care plans can also offer expanded care benefits. For example, in 1996, most Medicare HMOs offered one or more expanded services as part of their basic benefit package, such as routine physical examinations (97%), immunizations (86%), and outpatient drugs (60%) (Zarabozo, Taylor, & Hicks, 1996). Also common are vision exams (85%) and hearing exams (66%) (McMillan, 1993). Some plans offer a range from high to low benefit options with premiums varying by the optional benefits selected. Social/Health Maintenance Organizations are a special form of the risk model HMO.[3] These plans offer all the basic Medicare benefits indicated here, plus a limited set of chronic or long-term care benefits. These program benefits are discussed later in this chapter.

By 1996 about 13% of all Medicare beneficiaries were enrolled in managed care, with about 85% of these in risk contact plans. Medicare

---

[3] The authorization of S/HMO dates back to 1985, when Congress authorized a demonstration program that added community care benefits to a standard risk contract HMO. There are currently four plans in operation nationally.

risk contract enrollment increased by over 50% between 1994 and 1996, more than double the rate of growth in the non-Medicare sector. Twenty-five percent of the enrollment in Medicare risk HMOs occurs in five counties, but as of the beginning of 1996 only nine states did not have a Medicare risk HMO (two of these were served by out-of-state plans) (Zarabozo et al., 1996).

PRACTICES AND PERFORMANCE

Performance monitoring of managed care plans is an evolving endeavor. The most recent efforts reflect adaptations to the commercial sector's health maintenance organization performance measurement systems, more commonly known as HEDIS or Health Plan Employer Data Information Set. HEDIS was initially developed by the National Committee for Quality Assurance and the managed care industry as a performance measurement system. The initial measures included things like the percentage of children receiving immunizations and the percentage of age-appropriate women receiving mammographs. The list of measures is constantly expanding to include both processes of care and health outcomes. The growth in the number of measures or indicators is influenced by improvements in the completeness and accuracy of health plan information systems and a negotiated consensus on the importance of particular measures. Several initiatives are being pursued by the Health Care Financing Administration to influence these processes (Hadley & Wolfe, 1996). Among these are Medicare HEDIS (implemented in 1997); the Foundation for Accountability (FAcct), a public-private collaboration to develop outcome measures (first released in 1996); Quality Assurance Reform Initiative (QARI) a collaborative HCFA, state, industry, and consumer initiative to design and test practical approaches to Medicaid managed care service monitoring; Medicare Managed Care Quality Improvement Project, a pre-Medicare HEDIS effort to develop and test performance measures for use by peer review organizations (results released in 1997); and the HHS Interagency Managed Care Forum, meeting regularly to share information about managed care policy and other managed care activities.

Together these efforts, and those of the Joint Commission on Accreditation of Healthcare Organizations (JCAHO), represent an emerging approach to the conceptualization of access (cf., Docteur, Colby, & Gold, 1996) and quality-of-care monitoring systems (e.g., Friedman, 1995; Gagel, 1995; Jencks, 1995). The practical application of these systems is only just beginning. Because of this, much of what is known about managed care performance and practice has come from demonstration evaluations, national beneficiary surveys, or other focused studies. Some of this information is relatively dated, but materials have been selected because of their documentation of care access and the insights into the operational features of effective plan performance. Four major dimensions of care are reviewed: hospitals, physician, tests and procedures, home and skilled nursing.

Hospital Use

One of the principal ways HMOs have reduced their costs historically, relative to fee-for-service systems, is by controlling hospital admissions and lengths of stay. Prior to the advent of widespread managed care systems, and diagnosis related hospital reimbursement,[4] HMOs serving the non-Medicare population showed reductions of 10% to 40% in hospital days over fee-for-service indemnity reimbursed care. During the 1980s and early 1990s, studies have been less consistent in this finding. The Medical Outcomes Study found that HMO hospital utilization was 26% to 37% below FFS (Greenfield, Nelson, & Zubkoff, 1992). Other studies, including the Medicare risk contract evaluation, have shown either small differences (some with greater, others with fewer admission rates or lengths of stay) or statistically insignificant differences in admissions (cf., Miller & Luft, 1994a, 1997). These trends likely reflect the growing dominance of managed care over the hospital sector, and a convergence of practice patterns between fee-for-service and managed care providers. Among Medicare beneficiaries there was a 25% decline in fee-for-service hospital admissions per Medicare beneficiary between 1985 and 1989 as the delivery system adjusted to diagnostic-related reimbursement and the extension of outpatient care. During this period Medicare risk plans had between 6% to 9% fewer hospital days per beneficiary than did fee-for-service comparison groups (Brown & Hill, 1993). Admission and use rates varied among the various types of Medicare risk plans. Group and staff model plans had longer lengths of stay than IPA/network model

---

[4]Beginning in 1985, the Medicare program began a prospective payment system for hospitals based on a patient's diagnosis. This program reimburses the hospital a set amount for each of a set of diagnoses, regardless of the length of stay, and thus provides an incentive for hospitals to reduce lengths of stay. The extent and adverse effects of "earlier" discharge have been extensively studied by the Rand Corporation and others. An approximate doubling in the proportion of patients (i.e., 7% vs. 4%) discharged too soon or in an unstable condition, was found in the evaluations after PPS was initially implemented compared to prior to PPS (Kosecoff et al., 1990; Rubenstein et al., 1990). At the same time, unnecessarily lengthy stays diminished and the proportion of patients judged to be receiving "poor" or "very poor" care diminished from 25% to 12%.

plans. The S/HMO evaluation also found a lower use of hospitals relative to its fee-for-service comparison group after controlling for case mix (Newcomer, Manton, Harrington, Yordi, & Vertrees, 1995).

The relative effectiveness of managed care in reducing use and cost while reducing overtime is thought to be a consequence of tighter control on access to procedures, cost-saving incentives between the hospital and physicians (or between the physicians and the health plan) to reduce hospitalizations, and care protocols that shift some former hospital care into outpatient settings (cf., Conrad et al., 1996). Many of these factors are now relatively common in fee-for-service. The consequence of reduced hospital access and length of stay has been studied primarily in terms of rehospitalizations among those patients shifted to outpatient settings, and the functional performance of patients in these other levels of care.

Physician Use

The relative reduction in inpatient services within HMOs and managed care systems carries an implied assumption that physician or other services may have been expanded to accommodate a shift in care to an outpatient setting. There is no consistent empirical support for this. Of 24 studies reviewed by Miller and Luft (1994b, 1997), eight showed lower physician use (four were statistically significant) and eight with higher use (six were statistically significant). Complicating such comparisons is the parallel decline in inpatient days within the fee-for-service sector, and differences among the various managed care models. For example, in the Medical Outcomes Study, diabetic members had more (+9.1%) physician visits in group/staff model HMOs than in fee-for-service. Hypertensive HMO members had higher visits (+2%) in group/staff plans, while IPA members had fewer (−2%) visits (Greenfield, Rogers, Mangotich, Carney, & Tarlov, 1995). The Medicare risk contract evaluation also found substantially higher physician visit rates (19% to 25% more visits than fee-for-service) in staff/group models than network/IPA plans (with 3% fewer visits than fee-for-service) (Brown & Hill, 1993). A similar pattern was observed among S/HMOs (Newcomer et al., 1995).

More recent work has begun to examine what health plans are doing to affect clinical practice. The most widely used techniques are discounted fees and review of site of care, treatment appropriateness, and length of stay. Denial rates of recommended care generally were reported as being less than 3%. Primary care providers reported fewer denials than Medical specialists or surgeons. Rates were also higher in market areas where HMO penetration was higher (Remler et al., 1997). A second study has found no effect between how primary MDs are paid in managed care and the use of services (Conrad et al., 1998).

Tests and Procedures

Another presumed means of HMO savings is to use fewer services or to substitute less costly services when possible. Access to appropriate tests and procedures is both an important example of such cost controls, and a presumed indicator of the quality of care within health plans. There is some evidence that HMOs are economical in the use of tests and procedures, while still being attentive to prevention and health promotion. Findings from 14 studies (reviewed by Miller & Luft, 1994b, 1997), showed either better or equivalent access to tests and procedures. This was interpreted as indicating good quality of care. Included among these studies were six National Medicare Competition Evaluation analyses and two Medicare risk contract (or TEFRA HMO) evaluation studies. These studies generally showed that enrollees, whether Medicare beneficiaries or from group enrollment, were likely to receive the same or more frequent levels of routine and preventive care (such as cancer and hypertension screening tests; breast, pelvic, rectal, and general physical examinations) and to receive care similar to that received by nonenrollees for a variety of specific conditions. For example, analyses from the Medicare Competition Demonstration found that enrollees generally received tests and treatment comparable to nonenrollees for congestive heart failure, colorectal cancer, diabetes, and hypertension (Preston & Retchin, 1991; Retchin & Brown, 1990a, 1990b, 1991; Retchin & Preston, 1991). Similar findings were found in the treatment of stroke among Medicare Risk Contract plans (Retchin, Clement, & Brown, 1994) and rates of cancer screening with the Health Interview Survey (Bernstein, Thompson, & Harlan, 1991). However, two analysis of myocardial infarction showed that HMO enrollees had lower angiography and revascularization rates (Every, Fihn, Maynard, Martin, & Weaver, 1995; Langa & Sussman, 1993). Another study found that fee-for-service compliance with appropriateness guidelines exceed that of the HMOs for diagnostic testing (such as electrocardiograms and chest radiographs) (Carlisle et al., 1994).[5]

---

[5]The S/HMO demonstration evaluation approached the quality of care issue from a different perspective, using a comparison of changes in health status, life expectancy, and active life expectancy among plan members and those in fee-for-service. These results suggest generally comparable performance between the prepaid and indemnity systems among most health status groups, including the most frail. S/HMOs performance among females slightly trailed that of fee-for-service, but it was comparable among males (Manton, Newcomer, Vertrees, Lowrimore, & Harrington, 1993).

Another question with potential cost implications is whether managed care plans adopt innovative medical technology at rates comparable to fee-for-service systems. This issue has not been extensively studied, but one such investigation using gallbladder surgery techniques of laparoscopic cholecystomy as a illustrative comparison found no systematic difference between HMOs and fee-for-service in the acquisition of the technology (Chernew, Fendrick, & Hirth, 1997). Another study suggests that the more fundamental difference is not coverage, but in how use is controlled. Managed care entities typically set limits on the quantities of a service for which they will provide and pay. Fee-for-service coverage, on the other hand is typically unlimited, but with patient cost-sharing used as an incentive to limit utilization (Ramsey & Pauly, 1997).

Home Health and Skilled Nursing Care

Reductions in hospital admissions and days within managed care or other systems seemingly could be expected to increase nursing home and home health care use. However, Medicare patients in managed care, after adjusting for case mix, have been found to use about 15% fewer days of skilled nursing home care, and 20% fewer nurse or therapist visits (Brown & Hill, 1994). Two studies have found that HMO members get about 25% fewer home health aide visits than comparable cases using fee-for-service care (Brown & Hill, 1994; Shaughnessy, Schlenker, & Hittle, 1994). These results do not directly connect the use of these services to post-hospital care. Thus it is possible that hospital substitution occurs and that increases in post-hospital use are offset by reductions in admissions to home health and nursing homes for other cases. In a study specifically examining the effects of post-hospital care for Medicare patients, membership in an HMO had no significant effect on the likelihood of receiving various types of post-hospital care (Holtzman, Chen, & Kane, in press; Kane et. al., 1996). Comparisons between HMOs and fee-for-service should be interpreted in the context that managed care plans are financially at risk for home care skilled nursing, as well as hospital stays. Within the fee-for-service sector, hospitals are at risk for days of care, and thus have a greater incentive to shift patient care (and its associated financial risk) to other settings and providers.

Outcomes of home health care have been examined in terms of improvement and stabilization in functional status, mortality, discharge to independent living, and hospital utilization. After adjusting for case mix, Medicare fee-for-service patients, in at least one study, had better short-term outcomes relative to those in HMOs in measures of functionality (Shaughnessy et al., 1994). Among those with mild or moderate levels of impairment at "admission" to home health care, between 6% and 16% more fee-for-service patients improved in status than did the HMO counterparts over 12 weeks. However, there were no differences among those beginning with severe levels of disability. Similarly, there were no differences in the proportion discharged to independent living within 12 weeks, or in hospitalization within 12 weeks of start of care. This same study also conducted comparisons organized by rehabilitation and cardiac patients to assess home health service utilization differences for these high-risk groups. Fee-for-service patients received about one-third more total home health visits, and at least twice the number of home health aide visits and social service visits. There were, however, no significant differences in the number of skilled nursing, physical therapy, or occupational therapy visits for these conditions. Outcomes beyond 12 weeks were not measured in this study. The other study of Medicare post-hospital care (Kane et al., 1996) cited previously showed no differences in these longer-term outcomes for patients who were or were not HMO members.

The S/HMO demonstration, which included both Medicare reimbursed skilled nursing home and home health care benefits, and expanded benefits to cover nonskilled chronic care, provides some insight into the relationships between skilled and nonskilled services. Skilled nursing home use was highest in sites having the fewest hospital days per 1000 members. Home health days per 1000 also tended to be higher in these same sites, although the highest use of home health occurred among a high-use hospital site. Nonskilled nursing home use had no consistent relationship to skilled nursing days, nor was there a consistent relationship between nonskilled home care and either nursing home or home health care use (Harrington & Newcomer, 1991). The differences between plans was somewhat explained by organizational maturity (i.e., how long a plan had functioned as an HMO), and the financial risk relationship with their hospitals and medical groups. The more experienced organizations had lower use of high-cost services, and a tendency to substitute skilled care for these services. As a group the S/HMOs had more (9%–48%) hospital days per 1000 members than did the Medicare risk contract plans, and three times the skilled nursing and home health days of these plans. The rates for these latter services, controlling for case mix, approached those of the S/HMOs Medicare fee for service comparison group (Newcomer et al., 1995).

INTEGRATION OF ACUTE AND CHRONIC CARE SERVICES

Most managed care for older persons is offered as TEFRA HMOs, which cover only acute care. Even there, the prevailing model of health care and social service delivery, even within managed care systems, is one of compartmentalization. Physicians, usually the primary care physician, are responsible for outpatient care, while inpatient care is usually under the management of a medical specialist (e.g., surgeon, cardiologist, neurologist). Post-hospital skilled care, although "authorized" by a physician, is usually more directly managed by a nurse or therapeutic specialist (e.g., physical or occupational therapists). Nonskilled home care services, if not directly coordinated by the patient or a family member, are typically planned and monitored by a social services care manager (who may be a social worker). This latter process is most formalized in the home- and community-based programs financed through Medicaid and other state-administered programs.

The perspectives and scope of each of these multilevel approaches is influenced by the financing and reimbursement incentives associated with these levels of care, and by professional traditions. Historically, each level of care has operated within a compartmentalized budget and with its own treatment protocols. Under these arrangements, any cost savings from the substitution of lower for higher levels of care added cost to the programs financing lower-level services and produced savings for programs financing the higher levels of care. This structural feature, while long recognized, has generally not been well addressed, even in capitated managed care systems. The major exceptions to this within the Medicare and Medicaid programs are the Program for All Inclusive Care for the Elderly (PACE) which is a multi-site replication of the OnLok Senior Health Services program, the Social/Health Maintenance Organizations, Minnesota's Senior Health Options Program, Arizona's Health Care Cost Containment system (AHCCCS), and Arizona Long-Term Care System (ALTCS) systems discussed later. Risk contract HMOs have begun to implement various approaches to the identification and management of high-risk members. Several promising approaches to acute and chronic care integration are briefly described here, although their effectiveness has not yet been extensively evaluated.

Social/Health Maintenance Organization

The first generation of this Medicare demonstration, known as the S/HMO, was implemented in 1985 with the objective of adding a package of chronic care benefits to the acute services and operational structure of the Medicare HMO model. These chronic care benefits included unskilled nursing home stays (usually a maximum of 30 days), personal care, homemaker, and case management services. S/HMOs also offered expanded care benefits to all members, such as prescription drugs, eyeglasses, transportation, and preventive dental care. Two of the demonstration plans were established by mature HMOs: Kaiser Permanente Northwest in Portland, Oregon; and Group Health and Ebenezer Society developed a partnership in Minneapolis-St. Paul to establish Seniors Plus. Two S/HMOs were developed by long-term care organizations: the Metropolitan Jewish Geriatric Center established Elderplan; and Senior Health Action Network established SCAN Health Plan. (Group Health ceased offering its S/HMO plan in 1994.)

Among other purposes of the S/HMO demonstration was testing the efficacy of offering and managing access to chronic care benefits (e.g., non-skilled home care), and examining how the expansion of responsibility into community-based care affected the health plan's general approach to its aged members. The first-generation S/HMOs and the PACE demonstration differ in two fundamental ways. First, S/HMOs were targeted for the general Medicare population and competed directly with other Medicare risk-contract plans, whereas PACE is targeted at a specific, but small population: those older persons enrolled in both Medicare and Medicaid who are sufficiently frail to be eligible to be in nursing homes but are living in the community. Secondly, whereas PACE programs are responsible for the full range of acute and long-term care services, the S/HMOs' liability for chronic care to any individual member was capped (initially at an annual level of $6,000 to $12,000 depending on the plan), and did not extend to the long-term care liability of Medicaid coverage.

The first generation S/HMOs used a traditional model of outpatient and inpatient physician services and hospital utilization control. Each of these functions operated independently from the functional assessments, and chronic care benefit authorization and case management available to members. Contacts between physicians and case managers at all S/HMO sites were limited—usually to the authorization of Medicare services. Most physicians were uninvolved in chronic care plans and unaware when case management and chronic care services were provided to their patients. After 5 years of the demonstration, many S/HMO physicians were still unaware of the specific S/HMO benefits and when their patients were eligible for such services. S/HMO physicians generally did not utilize the resources of the case management staff, even for the most severely disabled patients.

Physician appointment schedules for S/HMO members were generally not adapted for patient age or complexity. The general failure of the plans to integrate and coordinate primary care and the management of high-risk cases is thought to be a contributing factor to the failure of these plans to experience lower annual costs for their very frail members and other case-mix groups than were observed among those in fee-for-service.[6] A related issue was that these plans were slow to develop treatment protocols or to use geriatricians, either as consultants to their primary care physicians or as primary care physicians themselves (Harrington, Lynch, & Newcomer 1993).

In 1995, the Health Care Financing Administration initiated the planning of a second generation model of the Social HMO. The second generation S/HMO demonstration retains the chronic care benefit package implemented in the first-generation plans, but it adds several fundamental refinements. Most important of these are an explicit attempt to develop a strong geriatric service model of care, and a reimbursement formula that is more directly tied to health care risk factors. The "geriatric" approach includes a screening program intended to identify patients at "risk" for high service costs and disability; timely application of primary care monitoring and treatment to reduce illness and disability; and a geriatric education and consultation program to provide specialty support for complex cases. Care management will support the primary care functions for those requiring home-based care, those discharged from hospitals or nursing homes, and those who are having difficulty complying with their treatment regimen. Case management efforts are closely integrated with the provision of primary care, including conferences among the various professionals. The proactive attention to clinical care and preventive services necessitates that the definition of "risk" includes acute and chronic conditions and problems, in addition to the limitations of activities of daily living which have been more typical in the long-term care field (Kane et al., 1997).[7]

These structural elements reflect current perspectives on how to integrate chronic care into an HMO. Such design changes are expected to solve the problems of fragmented health, social, and chronic care services for frail and disabled elders, and improve client outcomes and costs. The

---

[6]The S/HMOs generally experienced comparable or higher total expenditures for each of the six case mix groups formulated. These included healthy, acutely ill, IADL impaired, ADL impaired, cardiopulmonary, and very frail groups (Newcomer et al., 1995).

[7]The health plans selected for the planning phase of the demonstration were Fallon Community Health Plan, Worcester, Massachusetts; Health Plan of Nevada, Las Vegas, Nevada; Contra Costa County Health Plan, Martinez, California; Rocky Mountain HMO, Grand Junction, Colorado; CAC-Ramsay/United Health Plan, Dade County, Florida; Richland Memorial Hospital/Companion Health Care, Columbia, South Carolina. Health Plan of Las Vegas began enrolling members in October 1996 and had more than 25,000 S/HMO members by January 1998. Contra Costa Health Plan expects to begin enrolling members by the Winter of 1999. Rocky Mountain HMO is still officially active, but no start date has been set. None of the other plans are expected to become operational S/HMO plans, however, at least two states and one other health plan have requested approval from the Health Care Financing Administration to incorporate S/HMO reimbursement and operations in Medicare dually eligible programs.

biggest challenge to the plans is implementing effective coordination of primary care with case managers, geriatricians, other medical specialists, and long-term care providers. To date the major experience with comprehensive service integration has come from the staff model PACE program. There is little practical experience within network, independent practice associations, and general practice model HMOs on how best to do this.

Screening and Service Coordination in Medicare HMOs

The growth of managed care enrollment did not wait on the reported results from either the S/HMO or Medicare Risk Contract HMO evaluations. Studies of a selected group of the largest Medicare HMOs show that plans, as early as 1990, had begun to establish procedures for identifying high-risk patients, assessing and treating multi-problem patients, rehabilitating patients following acute events, reducing medication problems, and expanding benefits to include more home care and case management for nursing home patients (Kramer, Fox, & Morgenstern, 1992).

Screening, within the plans surveyed, was generally limited to new enrollees or hospital admissions, with an emphasis on physical functionality, cognitive status, medication use, and continence.[8] High-risk cases flagged via this process were referred to primary care (or geriatric assessment) for more in-depth assessments. Screening data were initially based on self-report questionnaires and telephone interviews. The screening of ongoing members appears to have been less formalized. It was generally based on an "informal referral" from the primary care physician, or triggered by hospitalization. A second survey of the largest Medicare HMOs 4 years later revealed that most plans were still not using their management information systems to identify high service-using members, or those with multiple chronic conditions—although this seems likely to occur soon, as management information systems are becoming more capable in capturing and reporting this information (Pacala et al., 1995).

The definition of "risk" has enlarged from that of the earlier S/HMO demonstrations, which was largely concerned with functional impairment and its implications for nursing home placement risk. Much more emphasis is given to health conditions and other factors that may be associated with hospitalization, preventable disability, and other avoidable expenditures.[9]

---

[8]This process varies somewhat from that of the S/HMO demonstration (both first and second generation plans) where annual reviews were made of all members and in-depth assessments were conducted among those with functional limitations.
[9]Much of this work has been influenced by Chad Boult and James Pacala and their associates (e.g., Pacala, Boult, & Boult, 1995; Pacala, Boult, Reed, & Aliberti, 1997) through the development of the PRA, or Probability of Repeated Admission. The dimensions and measures used in this and related screening and assessment instruments have a low false positive rate when identifying high-

Follow-up patient assessments (within the group of plans surveyed in 1990) were, at least in theory, conducted by a team consisting of a geriatrician, nurse practitioner, and social worker. Primary care for post-acute care patients was done by a combination of methods (Kramer et al., 1992). For those returning home, most plans relied on the primary care physician. For persons in skilled nursing homes, some plans relied on the primary care physician, others had a medical director who handled all such cases, and still others used a nurse practitioner for primary care. Combinations of these approaches may have occurred depending on whether the nursing home was a primary referral site for the health plan or free-standing facility with only a few plan members. The management of other "high-risk," but not hospitalized, cases apparently largely fell on the primary care physician. In most of the plans, a nurse practitioner may have provided primary care to long-stay nursing home residents.

The effectiveness of these approaches within each of the health plans has not been formally reported, but experience from clinical trials and other studies informs expectations of program success. The dissemination of program innovations and refinements is occurring rapidly among health plans, both through their national trade association, the Group Health Association of America, and rapidly growing specialty organizations, such as the National Chronic Care Consortium. These consortia were formed by health plans specifically to exchange information on "state of the art" products and on their experience with service integration across the continuum of outpatient to inpatient, and between acute and chronic care (Fama, Fox, & White, 1995).

Geriatricians and Multi-disciplinary Teams

The extent that geriatric medicine should and can be integrated into the delivery of managed care is not yet resolved. Geriatricians can be used in several ways in managed care settings (Friedman & Kane, 1993). Historically, some HMOs have used geriatricians as part of their primary care practitioner group, but without allowing these physicians to limit their practice exclusively to geriatric patients.

---

cost patients, but they miss substantial portions of the true positives (i.e., those with high cost). Further work is ongoing by this group, those involved in planning the second generation S/HMO, and others to more efficiently identify those at risk of high cost. Further work is especially needed on how to link screening information with treatment protocols. A further impetus for such measurement work is the desire to develop risk adjusted capitation reimbursement. Work by Hornbrook and Goodman, 1996, Manton et al., 1994, and others has shown the predictive value of combining functional ability, chronic conditions, and demographic factors in estimating health care expenditures.

Another model for practice is to have geriatricians (or a geriatric team) provide care and management to the most frail and vulnerable elderly within a system. This is implemented through screening programs, such as those noted earlier, that identify and refer new members who are frail (or those members who have become frail) into this specialty practice for ongoing primary care. Such a model requires a large elderly enrollment to generate cost-effective practice volume. A variant on this model uses geriatricians as specialist consultants for assessment and advice with ongoing treatment. The patient remains under the care of their regular primary care physician. These two models can also be used in combination.

A further variation on the above involves the use of multidisciplinary teams (i.e., nurses, social workers, and/or other health professionals) to augment the primary care physician. This model recognizes that geriatric training is generally more common among nurses and social workers, and it allows for case monitoring to occur through means other than office visits and to encompass care plans that go beyond purely medical treatment. In many cases, geriatric nurse practitioners (GNPs) or adult nurse practitioners (ANPs) might assume responsibility for basic primary care, freeing the geriatrician's time for more complex cases. These team models can be for ambulatory care operating as components in ambulatory care clinics, or as adjuncts to the home care program. Such teams, as discussed earlier, are perhaps even more common in hospital inpatient, and nursing home settings. Under these inpatient circumstances the team likely replaces the patient's primary care physician, until the patient returns to the community.

One area where GNPs have been used to good advantage is in providing primary care to nursing home patients. A corporation, Evercare, has developed a cost-effective managed care approach to capitating the acute care of nursing home patients, using GNPs as the major source of the more intensive than usual primary care. The underlying premise of this approach is that closer attention to the nursing home residents' primary care needs will reduce the use of more expensive hospital care (Polich, Bayard, Jacobson, & Parker, 1990). EverCare is being demonstrated in six sites across the country. As it has been implemented, some changes have been necessary. The participating physicians are recruited from those in the community already active in nursing home care. Because sufficient numbers of geriatric nurse practitioners are not always available, adult nurse practitioners are sometimes used instead.

The relative value of any of these approaches is largely untested, but as a practical matter, the choices made by a health plan are constrained by the size of the Medicare enrollment, and the availability of geriatricians over the short term. There are currently relatively few geriatric medicine specialists available in the U.S. Approximately 8,400 MDs were board certified in geriatrics in the U.S. between 1988 (when the exam was initiated) and 1994 (American Geriatrics Society, 1995).[10]

Regardless of the practice approach, a major interest of the plans is minimizing inappropriate hospitalization and emergency room visits. In addition to the use of geriatric teams for primary and specialty care, regular care monitoring by telephone calls, home visits from case management units, and 24-hour advice from nurse services are becoming common. The criteria triggering a patient into such surveillance, the frequency of the monitoring, and the mechanisms of information coordination among the physician and the case management units are still being refined. The functional form of this communication and the incentives affecting participation are somewhat affected by the services involved.

Such relationships are illustrated by hospital discharge planning, perhaps the best developed example of case management activity. When the hospital is not owned and/or operated by the managed care plan, discharge planners may have a stronger incentive to be efficient in carrying out their activities, since the plan is incurring billable expenses. Similarly, the planners may be less likely to consider rehabilitation units, subacute, or SNF units if these are not owned by the plan. Alternatively, these services may be used as substitutes for hospital care. Further complicating these relationships is coordination between hospital discharge planners and other case managers/or care coordinators. Even if both are employed by the managed care plan, there still may be conflicts because of difference(s) in how each unit interprets patient needs and organizational goals.

While issues such as this, and case management more generally, have not been systematically studied in managed health plans, the outcomes of the discharge planning process have generally focused on reducing the hospital readmission rates, reducing ER visits and reductions in posthospital complications. One key to improved outcomes is that the individuals discharged be in a stable condition, an issue discussed earlier in this chapter.

Clinical Practice Guidelines

The Institute of Medicine (IoM) defines clinical practice guidelines as "systematically developed statements to assist practitioner and patient

---

[10]In the first generation S/HMOs, few geriatric physicians were available in the SHMOs, and when available, they were required to carry full patient loads and could not limit their practices to geriatrics. Additionally, none of the sites tested either a geriatric assessment or multidisciplinary team approach to providing medical care to the frail elderly. Furthermore, frail elderly were not routinely assigned to physicians with geriatric training or geriatric nurses. Where nurse practitioners were utilized (at one site), it was for nursing home patients only (Harrington et al., 1993).

decisions about appropriate health care for specific clinical circumstances" (Field & Lohr, 1992, p. 27). The American Medical Association and medical specialty societies appear to prefer the term "practice parameters." Other terms, such as practice standards, protocols, and appropriateness indicators, are also commonly used in the literature and practice. However labeled, practice guidelines have existed in a variety of forms for some time. It is estimated that several thousand "guideline-like" statements and documents have been produced by different medical societies, and by associations for other care professions.

The federal government, until recently, was also active in this effort. Most prominent was the Agency for Health Care Policy and Research (AHCPR), whose Forum on Quality and Effectiveness in Health Care operated between 1990 and 1997. Through 1995, the forum had produced 15 complete guidelines and had many in development.[11] Other agencies involved in guideline development include the National Institutes of Health through its consensus development conference program in the NIH Office of Medical Applications of Research; the Centers for Disease Control and Prevention; the US Preventive Services Task Force; the Health Care Financing Administration; and the congressional Office of Technology Assessment. Together these agencies produce many more guidelines than AHCPR.

Private research organizations such as the Rand Corporation; academic health centers; physician specialty societies; numerous health plans and provider groups, payers and insurers, such as Blue Cross and Blue Shield; and other entities, such as pharmaceutical companies, have also produced guidelines. Some of these are for research applications. Others are to help with internal quality assurance. Such guidelines number in the thousands, and are growing; their volume raises questions about having so many versions of the truth.

At their most basic level, guidelines are checklists of tests or procedures that should be considered in the presence of a specific health problem or

---

[11] Guidelines published through 1995 include the following topics: acute pain management; urinary incontinence in adults; prediction, prevention, and treatment of pressure ulcers in adults; management of functional impairment due to cataracts; depression in primary care; sickle cell disease; evaluation and management of early infection with HIV; diagnosis and treatment of benign prostatic hyperplasia; management of cancer pain; diagnosis and management of unstable angina; evaluation and care of heart failure; otitis media with effusion in young children; quality determinants of mammography; acute low back problems in adults. Topics with expected 1996 release dates include: post-stroke rehabilitation, cardiac rehabilitation, recognition and initial assessment of Alzheimer's and related dementias, smoking prevention and cessation, and an update of urinary incontinence in adults. The last guidelines developed were those related to panic disorder, osteoporosis, and early detection of breast cancer. The negative response to the AHCPR guidelines from some organizations created a political problem. The AHCPR has now shifted its strategy to develop systematic studies of effectiveness without translating these into guidelines. Guidelines will be published as a book in 1999.

condition. The guidelines of highest quality are based on a combination of scientific-based evidence and clinical judgment. Guidelines produced in the absence of a research base of outcome studies usually reflect substantial effort at clinical judgment consensus.

Expectations about the utility of practice guidelines in improving appropriateness of care, reducing the number of unnecessary tests or procedures, and reducing expenditures, run high—at least among proponents. Success in achieving these expectations is dependent on several fundamental conditions. Perhaps the most basic condition is sufficiency of scientific evidence upon which to base guidelines. According to the IoM guidelines report (Field & Lohr, 1992), the scientific evidence for efficacious treatment is strong for about 4% of all health services. For about 45% of patient care the scientific evidence is modest, but with a high level of clinical consensus. For the balance of areas there is a weak or nonexistent scientific basis (although again, agreement among clinicians may be high).

Limitations such as these may retard the use of guidelines by practitioners or, even if used faithfully, the clinical outcomes achieved may not be as efficacious as expected. The dearth of empirical information can be solved with greatly expanded efforts at outcomes and effectiveness research, and more attention to clinical evaluation. Improvements in the scientific basis of guidelines is by itself not sufficient, however. The proliferation of guidelines and their varied rigor pose problems in the choice of which guidelines to adopt, quality control over content, conflicting or inconsistent practice recommendations and, ultimately, acceptance by practitioners. A study by the American College of Physicians (ACP) reported that their members gave ACP-developed guidelines a confidence rating of 82%. This contrasted to a 6% rating given to Blue Cross and Blue Shield guidelines (Tunis et al., 1994). Confidence ratings aside, there remain additional concerns about the timeliness of the information in the guidelines, how this is updated, and the qualifications of those who interpret them. This latter concern is thought to be particularly troublesome when insurers or health plans use guidelines for treatment authorization and utilization control (Parker, 1995).

Is there any empirical evidence to show that guidelines achieve the expected results in modifying practice patterns, the quality of care, and cost reductions? This question is best answered by distinguishing between guidelines applied with sanctions and those without; and with the caveat that few of the myriad guidelines have actually been studied. In other words, what is known in this area is based on a limited number of practice guidelines. Few of the studies are specific to geriatrics (Grimshaw & Russell, 1993; Lomas, Sisk, & Stocking, 1993). Information- or education-only guidelines (usually in the form of continuing education or clinical trial result reporting) generally do not seem to produce changes in practice (Davis, Thompson, Oxman, & Haynes, 1992). To make practice standards more effective it seems helpful to combine them with some other influence—such as participation of the physician in their development, promulgation by opinion leaders, and feedback of practice patterns. In these respects, the limited work reported to date finds that clinical trial results from drug studies are associated with practice behavior (Lamas et al., 1992). Guidelines not based on clinical trial data are much less effective in changing behavior (Lomas et al., 1993), as are guidelines (including NIH consensus panel work) that are distributed without much publicity or organizational endorsement (Kosecoff et al., 1987).

When guidelines are publicized with appropriate practitioners, and backed by assurances from opinion leaders that quality will not be compromised and that cost savings are substantial, then behavior does seem to be affected (Pauly, 1995). Comparisons of practice profiles and feedback on monitoring of bad outcomes also seem to change behavior (Mugford, Banfield, & O'Hanlon, 1991).

Studies of guidelines having an explicit monetary sanction for deviations are very limited. This occurs in some measure because of the general absence of such systems, even in managed care organizations. Perhaps the best example of this type of sanction is represented by physician response to the Medicare DRG reimbursement. The reduction in hospital length of stay as this program was phased in has been suggested as indicating that physicians were influenced to follow hospital and medical staff guidelines about lengths of stay and discharge (Pauly, 1995). Similar patterns have been discussed in preceding sections with respect to physician behavior in managed care systems more generally. In those situations, physician behavior may be tied as much to the financial incentive of sharing in hospital cost savings as to actual sanctions.

Managed care organizations and their associated providers have both a professional and ethical interest in avoiding the provision of inappropriate care. Similarly, they have an organizational interest in avoiding unnecessary expenditures. As managed care systems attempt to strengthen utilization controls, it is likely that these dual objectives may come into conflict. This is an important area for further study. It is one that has yet to receive much empirical attention.

Medicaid

Many federal agencies, state governments, providers, and foundations are interested in using managed care as a vehicle for integrating acute care and LTC (long-term care). The goal of such integration is widely endorsed, however there are a number of unresolved practical questions. Two of the most important of these are discussed here.

First, combining acute care and LTC under the aegis of a single entity raises some important questions about auspices. Many proponents of LTC fear that such a merged authority will be dominated by a medical mentality, and that important attributes of LTC will receive short shrift. A second issue has to do with the knowledge and experience base upon which to establish payment rates. Most state long-term care programs can be characterized by adjusting Medicaid payments based on expected Medicare reimbursement. Contractors in these situations are responsible for actually obtaining the Medicare portion. If Medicaid is capitated, Medicare usually remains fee-for-service—creating an incentive to shift costs to the fee-for-service payer. If acute care for both Medicaid and Medicare is capitated then usually LTC is fee-for-service—creating no incentive for capitated plans to keep members out of the LTC system because Medicaid will pay for long-term chronic stays. Data systems that can accumulate the full cost (across both Medicare and Medicaid) of the LTC population or those at risk of entering the LTC system are only beginning to be implemented. And importantly, available data are affected by the incentives that influenced the choice of care within segregated delivery models.

Recognizing these important knowledge gaps, it is not surprising that states have approached integration in an incremental manner. A handful of states (Arizona, California, Florida, Massachusetts, Minnesota, Ohio, and Wisconsin) have enrolled elderly persons into Medicaid managed care programs that include varying levels of LTC. These are briefly profiled below. A common characteristic of all these programs to date is that none includes a direct role for the state regarding Medicare reimbursement.

Arizona

Arizona is the only state with a statewide managed care program for persons needing LTC (Arizona Long Term Care System, or ALTCS). It has not yet integrated Medicare coverage. The Arizona Health Care Cost Containment system (AHCCCS) contracts with managed care organizations (MCOs) for the coverage of all Medicaid enrollees. Medicaid recipients are enrolled in ALTCS only if they meet the LTC criteria measured by Arizona's preadmission screening tool. Through ALTCS, the state pays contractors (private MCOs in the Phoenix and Tucson areas and counties themselves in the larger, less populous counties) a capitated rate that covers the full range of community-based LTC and nursing home care. ALTCS contractors are also responsible for the primary and acute care needs of their members. In the larger, less populous counties, ALTCS services are provided directly by the county-operated programs. Client care is coordinated in an effort to integrate the acute care and LTC; however, at present this program covers only Medicaid costs, with Medicare costs still reimbursed on a fee-for-service basis. Negotiations are underway to include Medicare in the managed care arrangement.

Wisconsin

The Wisconsin Partnership Program serves persons eligible for nursing facilities in small programs that have incorporated interdisciplinary care management. The program currently operates as a Medicaid prepaid health plan (which is partially capitated). Medicare is billed by the providers on a fee-for-service basis at present. However, program planners intend to seek federal approval for full capitation of both Medicaid and Medicare services.

Florida

Florida has undertaken demonstration projects in three counties with two participating MCOs to examine the effects of managed Medicaid programs for seniors. Only recipients who meet the state's preadmission screening for nursing home eligibility are eligible, and during the demonstration phase only those age 65 and older were eligible.

In these projects, only Medicaid is capitated (similar to the Arizona ALTCS program). Moreover, by state law, the lead MCOs in the demonstration are prohibited from enrolling the members in a Medicare risk contract. The benefits include a variety of in-home services, including in-home care, day care, escort services, supplies, and home adaptations. Case management is an important feature of the program, and is particularly necessary for enrollees receiving acute care.

Minnesota

Minnesota's Prepaid Medical Assistance Program (PMAP) enrolls elderly persons and does include some community-based LTC and limited nursing facility care (up to 90 days), but it pays for additional LTC on a fee-for-service basis. Minnesota has initiated an §1115 waiver to establish the *Senior Health Options Project (MSHO)*, which integrates a full range of Medicare and Medicaid services for older persons who are dually eligible, regardless of whether they need LTC. Nursing facility liability will be limited to 180 days, but the rate structure will provide incentives to provide community care.

Mixed Capitation and FFS Programs

Other state programs include some community-based LTC services within a capitation but that continue to pay for other LTC services (notably nursing home stays) on a fee-for-service basis. This is true of Wisconsin's "I Care" Program (serving persons with disabilities ages 15 and up) and of Ohio's Accessing Better Care (ABC) program (limited to persons with disabilities under age 65). In those programs, enhanced community-based services are part of the benefit package, but persons are disenrolled if they enter a nursing facility.

CONCLUSIONS

The transformation of the health care delivery system toward managed care raises both alarms and opportunities. Those who view the current managed care organization (MCO) growth as an express train are understandably concerned that the emphasis seems to be on pricing, evidenced by the Balanced Budget Act's focus on price reduction. There are large profits and Medicare savings to be made in controlling the costs of what has become a bloated health care system. This first wave of MCOs can be thought of as the Wal-Mart era. It is characterized by high-volume purchasing of recognized services on the basis of discounted rates.

A more hopeful scenario looks toward a second generation of MCOs, when discounting will have achieved its full competitive role and competition will be based on real efficiencies. This era may be thought of as the information age of MCOs. Here the emphasis will be placed on enhanced coordination and more effective care for the elderly.

The early experience of Medicare risk contract HMOs, the Social/Health Maintenance Organizations, and the PACE demonstration sites all show evidence of at least comparable care outcomes to those of fee-for-service delivery. Though such findings are encouraging, they should be viewed in the context that they have been obtained from organizations willing to participate in national demonstrations and complex evaluation research designs. The persistence of the performance achieved by these programs over time, and the achievement of comparable performance by the myriad of managed care plans expanding into new market areas, are issues requiring ongoing monitoring.

An empirical reminder of this comes from a Medical Outcomes Study analysis of aged persons with chronic health conditions. Relatively poorer health status outcomes were found after 4 years for HMO members compared to similar persons in fee-for-service (Ware, Bayliss, Rogers, Kosinski, & Tarlov, 1996). The hypothesized explanation for this finding was a possible "S" shape to the relationship between health care access and outcomes. Under this hypothesis, outcomes on the top and flatter portion of the curve are relatively unaffected by reductions in expenditures because health outcome benefits no longer improve with marginal increases in expenditures. Outcomes on the steep portion of the curve are much more sensitive to expenditure levels. Such work, while not definitive (and in conflict with many prior Medical Outcome Study findings), suggests that the need for access to care likely varies among patient subgroups, including those with chronic conditions. (For additional thoughts on this issue see Wagner, 1997; Riley, Tudor, Chiang, & Ingber, 1996.)

Another explanation for the contradiction between this recent MOS finding and the preponderance of the other prior work may be suggested by disenrollments from HMOs. Historically, Medicare beneficiaries could change plans monthly if they so elected. This was a built-in assurance of their ability to obtain care. Most demonstration studies of Medicare HMO members have found comparably high levels of health care satisfaction among HMO members and those in fee-for-service (e.g., Rossiter, Langwell, Wang, & Rivnyak, 1989). This has also been observed in analyses of the Medicare Current Beneficiary Survey, a probability sample of beneficiaries (Lee & Kasper, 1998). Satisfaction has been found to be relatively lower among persons with functional disability, even in plans having special programs for these populations (Newcomer, Preston, & Harrington, 1996). The ability to leave may have masked dissatisfaction about the level of care available to them. One study comparing fee-for-service use among persons disenrolling from HMOs with similar persons who had been on in fee-for-service care found substantially higher rates of service and expenditures among those leaving HMOs (Morgan, Virning, DeVito, & Persily, 1997). When utilization rates returned to the prevailing levels among fee-for-service members, the former HMO members had a tendency to return to the HMOs. As Medicare policy changes to require HMO enrollment on an annual basis, the previously observed levels of satisfaction and comparable health care outcomes may decline if the plans do not adjust to the needs and expectations of those with chronic conditions.

Certainly incentives exist within capitation financing for a balance between the service rationing needed to control costs, and the proactive care needed to assure desirable quality-of-care outcomes. Many models or approaches to the identification of "at risk" patients, the delivery of primary care, and ongoing monitoring and management of complex patient care are emerging (e.g., Boult, Pacala, & Boult, 1995). These will be refined with experience and the exchange of this experience among health plans. No single approach seems likely to dominate, as these are potentially affected by the size of the plan's membership, the supply of competing alternative services within a service area, and the components of the delivery system owned by the managed care plan (or its participating providers). Consolidation of managed care plans, consolidation between medical groups and hospitals, and formalized arrangements between managed care organizations and long-term care providers are but some of the delivery system elements in transition even as Medicare beneficiary participation in managed care grows more generally. Thus, there is reason for optimism in the mid-term about the effectiveness of managed care; and reason for concern in the short term as approaches are tried, and organizational effectiveness is tested.

Combining or integrating acute care and LTC raises some important questions about whether the merged authority will be dominated by a medical mentality and the cost-saving incentives which these entities will experience. There is concern among many that LTC will receive short shrift, to the extent that acute care and LTC address somewhat different goals. Much of LTC can be said to be based on a compensatory approach, wherein functional deficits are met by services that the clients can no longer provide for themselves. Acute care has historically had a more curative bent, seeking to change a client's status rather than cope with it. On the other hand, there is a basis for optimism even if medical entities do dominate the delivery systems. As emphasis in medical care has shifted from infectious disease to chronic disease, appreciation of the need to address the patient in a larger life context has also grown. Issues related to quality of life are also increasingly recognized and addressed.

HCFA's (and the managed care industry's) quality-of-care monitoring systems are adapting to these changing delivery systems, but they will not be online for several years. In the meanwhile, other evaluative systems will be needed. Additionally, mechanisms for testing and refining important elements of the managed care delivery models are needed. Among the immediately available resources for doing this are the second generation of the Social/Health Maintenance Organization demonstrations, PACE, and the state managed care programs among long-term care populations. An important feature of all these programs is an explicit attempt to develop a strong geriatric service model of care, and a reimbursement formula that is more directly tied to health care risk factors. The "geriatric" approach includes a screening program intended to identify patients at "risk" for high service costs and disability; timely application of primary care monitoring and treatment to reduce illness and disability; and a geriatric education and consultation program to provide specialty support for complex cases. Care management supports the primary care functions for those requiring home based care, those discharged from hospitals or nursing homes, and those who are having difficulty complying with their treatment regimens. The proactive attention to clinical care and preventive services necessitates that the definition of "risk" include acute and chronic conditions and problems, in addition to the limitations of activities of daily living which have been more typical in the long-term care field.

These structural elements reflect current perspectives on how to integrate chronic care into an HMO. Such design changes are expected to solve the problems of fragmented health, social, and chronic care services for frail and disabled elders, and improve client outcomes and costs. The biggest challenge to the plans is implementing effective coordination of primary care with case managers, geriatricians, other medical specialists, and long-term care providers. To date, the major experience with comprehensive service integration has come from the staff model PACE program. There is little practical experience within networks, independent practice associations, and general practice model HMOs on how to best do this.

Medicaid programs are rapidly developing managed care plans for their non-elderly recipients. Medicare beneficiary enrollment into managed care plans will also continue. Research and demonstration efforts, whether financed by the government, foundations, or private corporations, are needed to test the efficacy of service integration approaches, and other refinements in the delivery of care.

REFERENCES

American Geriatrics Society. (1995). *Statistics on board certified physicians in geriatrics.* New York: American Geriatric Society.

Armstead, R., Elstein, P., & Gorman, J. (1995). Toward a 21st century quality-measurement system for managed-care organizations. *Health Care Financing Review, 16,* 25–37.

Bernstein, A., Thompson, G., & Harlan, L. (1991). Differences in rates of cancer screening by usual source of medical care: Data from the 1987 National Health Interview Survey. *Medical Care, 29,* 196–209.

Boult, C., Pascala, J., & Boult, L. (1995). Targeting elders for geriatric evaluation and management: Reliability, validity, and practicality of a questionnaire. *Aging, 7,* 159–164.

Brown, R., & Hill, J. (1993). *Does model type play a role in the extent of HMO effectiveness in controlling the utilization of services?* Princeton, NJ: Mathematica Policy Research.

Brown, R., & Hill, J. (1994). The effects of Medicare risk HMOs on Medicare costs and service utilization. In H. Luft (Ed.), *HMOs and the elderly* (pp. 13–49). Ann Arbor, MI: Health Administration Press.

Carlisle, D., Siu, A., Keeler, E., Kahn, K., Rubenstein, L., & Brook, R. (1994). Do HMOs provide better care for older patients with acute myocardio infarction? In H. Luft (Ed.), *HMOs and the elderly* (pp. 195–214). Ann Arbor, MI: Health Administration Press.

Chernew, M., Fendrick, A., & Hirth, R. (1997). Managed care and medical technology: Implications for cost growth. *Health Affairs, 16*, 196–206.

Conrad, D., Maynard, C., Cheadle, A., Ramsey, S., Marcussmith, M., Kirz, H., Madden, C., Martin, D., Perrin, E., Wickizer, T., Zierler, B., Ross, A., Noren, J., & Liang, S. (1998). Primary care physician compensation method in medical groups—does it influence the use and cost of health services for enrollees in managed care organizations. *JAMA, 279*(11), 853–858.

Conrad, D., Noren, J., Marcus-Smith, M., Ramsey, S., Kirz, H., Wickizer, T., Perrin, E., & Ross, A. (1996). Physician compensation models in medical group practice. *Journal of Ambulatory Care Management, 19*, 18–27.

Conrad, D., Wickizer, T., Maynard, C., Klastorin, T., Lessler, D., Ross, A., Soderstrom, N., Sullivan, S., Alexander, J., & Travis, K. (1996). Managing care, incentives, and information: An exploratory look inside the "black box" of hospital efficiency. *Health Services Research, 31*, 235–260.

Davis, D., Thompson, M., Oxman, A., & Haynes, R. (1992). Evidence for effectiveness of CME: A review of 50 randomized controlled trials. *Journal of the American Medical Association, 268*, 1111–1117.

Docteur, E., Colby, D., & Gold, M. (1996). Shifting the paradigm: Monitoring access in Medicare managed care. *Health Care Financing Review, 17*, 5–22.

Every, N., Fihn, S., Maynard, C, Martin, J., & Weaver, W. (1995). Resource utilization in treatment of acute myocardial infarction: Staff-model health maintenance organization versus fee-for-service hospitals. *Journal of the American College of Cardiology, 26*, 401–406.

Fama, T., Fox, P., & White, L. (1995). Do HMOs care for the chronically ill? *Health Affairs, 14*, 234–243.

Field, M., & Lohr, K. (Eds.). (1992). *Guidelines for clinical practice: From development to use.* Washington, DC: National Academy Press.

Friedman, M. (1995). Issues in measuring and improving health care quality. *Health Care Financing Review, 16*, 1–13.

Friedman, B., & Kane, R. (1993). HMO medical director's perceptions of geriatric practice in Medicare HMOs. *Journal of the American Geriatric Society, 41*, 1144–1149.

Gagel, B. (1995). Health care quality improvement program: A new approach. *Health Care Financing Review, 16*, 15–23.

Greenfield, S., Nelson, E., & Zubkoff, M. (1992). Variations in resource utilization among medical specialties and systems of care: Results from the Medical Outcomes Study. *Journal of the American Medical Association, 267*, 1624–1630.

Greenfield, S., Rogers, W., Mangotich, M., Carney, M., & Tarlov, A. (1995). Outcomes of patients with hypertension and non insulin dependent diabetes mellitus treated by different systems and specialties: Results from the Medical Outcomes Study. *Journal of the American Medical Association, 274*, 1436–1444.

Grimshaw, J., & Russell, I. (1993). Effects of clinical guidelines on medical practice: A systematic review of rigorous evaluations. *Lancet, 342*, 1317–1322.

Hadley, J., & Wolfe, L. (1996). Monitoring and evaluating the delivery of services under managed care. *Health Care Financing Review, 17*, 1–4.

Harrington, C., Lynch, M., & Newcomer, R. (1993). Medical services in social health maintenance organizations. *The Gerontologist, 33*, 790–800.

Harrington, C., & Newcomer, R. (1991). Social health maintenance organization service use and costs, 1985–1989. *Health Care Financing Review, 12*, 37–52.

Holtzman, J., Chen, Q., & Kane, R. (1998). The effect of HMO status on the outcomes of home care following hospitalization in a Medicare population. *Journal of the American Geriatrics Society, 46*, 629–634.

Hornbrook, M., & Goodman, M. (1996). Chronic disease, functional health status, and demographics: A multi-dimensional approach to risk adjustment. *Health Services Research, 31*, 283–308.

Jencks, S. (1995). Measuring quality of care under Medicare and Medicaid. *Health Care Financing Review, 16*, 39–54.

Jenson, G., Morrisey, M., Gaffney, S., & Liston, D. (1997). The new dominance of managed care: Insurance trends in the 1990s. *Health Affairs, 16*, 125–136.

Kane, R., Finch, M., Blewett, L., Chen, Q., Burns, R., & Moskowitz, M. (1996). Use of post-hospital care by Medicare patients. *Journal of the American Geriatrics Society, 44*, 242–250.

Kane, R. L., & Friedman, B. (1997). State variations in Medicare expenditures. *American Journal of Public Health, 87*, 1611–1619.

Kane, R. L., Kane, R. A., Finch, M., Harrington, C., Newcomer, R., Miller, N., & Hulbert, M. (1997). S/HMOs, the second generation: Building on the experience of the first Social Health Maintenance Organization demonstrations. *Journal of the American Geriatrics Society, 45*, 101–107.

Kosecoff, J., Kahn, K., Rogers, W., Reinisch, E., Sherwood, M., Rubenstein, L., Draper, P., Roth, C., Chew, C., & Brook, R. (1990). Prospective payment system and impairment at discharge: The "quicker-and-sicker" story revisited. *Journal of the American Medical Association, 264*, 1980–1983.

Kosecoff, J., Kanouse, D., Rogers, W., McCloskey, L., Winslow, C., & Brook, R. (1987). Effects of the National Institutes of Health Consensus Development Program on physician practice. *Journal of the American Medical Association, 258*, 2708–2713.

Kramer, A., Fox, P., & Morgenstern, N. (1992). Geriatric care approaches in health maintenance organizations. *Journal of the American Geriatrics Society, 40*, 1055–1067.

Lamas, G., Pfeffer, M., Hamm, P., Wertheimer, J., Rousleau, J., & Braunwald, E. (1992). Do the results of randomized clinical trials of cardiovascular drugs influence medical practice? *New England Journal of Medicine, 327*, 241–274.

Langa, K., & Sussman, E. (1993). The effects of cost containment policies on rates of coronary revascularization in California. *The New England Journal of Medicine, 329,* 1784–1789.

Lee, Y., & Kasper, J. (1998). Assessment of medical care by elderly people: General Satisfaction and physician quality. *Health Services Research, 32,* 741–758.

Lomas, J., Sisk, J., & Stocking, B. (1993). From evidence to practice in the United States, the United Kingdom, and Canada. *Milbank Quarterly, 71,* 405–410.

Manton, K., Newcomer, R., Lowrimore, G., Vertrees, J., & Harrington, C. (1993). Social/health maintenance organization and fee for service health outcomes overtime. *Health Care Financing Review, 15,* 173–202.

Manton, K., Newcomer, R., Vertrees, J., Lowrimore, G., & Harrington, C. (1994). A method for adjusting capitation payments to managed care plans using multivariate patterns of health and functioning: The experience of the social/health maintenance organizations. *Medical Care, 32,* 277–297.

McMillan, A. (1993). Trends in Medicare health maintenance organization enrollment: 1986–1993. *Health Care Financing Review, 15,* 135–146.

Miller, R., & Luft, H. (1994b). Managed care plans: Characteristics, growth, and premium performance. *Annual Review of Public Health, 15,* 437–459.

Miller, R., & Luft, H. (1994a). Managed care plan performance since 1980: A literature analysis. *Journal of the American Medical Association, 271,* 1512–1519.

Miller, R., & Luft, H. (1997). Does managed care lead to better or worse quality of care? A survey of recent studies shows mixed results on managed care plan performance. *Health Affairs, 16,* 7–25.

Morgan, R., Virning, B., DeVito, C., & Persily, N. (1997). The Medicare-HMO revolving door: The healthy go in and the sick go out. *New England Journal of Medicine, 337,* 169–175.

Mugford, M., Banfield, P., & O'Hanlon, M. (1991). Effects of feedback of information on clinical practice: A review. *British Medical Journal, 3003,* 398–402.

Newcomer, R., Manton, K., Harrington, C., Yordi, C., & Vertrees, J. (1995). Case mix controlled service use and expenditures in the social health maintenance organization demonstration. *Journal of Gerontology: Medical Sciences, 50a,* M35–M44.

Newcomer, R., Preston, S., & Harrington, C. (1996) Health plan satisfaction, functional frailty, and risk of disenrollment from Social/HMOs. *Inquiry, 33,* 144–154.

Pacala, J., Boult, C., & Boult, L. (1995). Predictive validity of a questionnaire that identifies older persons at risk for hospital admission. *Journal of the American Geriatrics Society, 43,* 374–377.

Pacala, J., Boult, C., Hepburn, K., Kane, R., Kane, R., Malone, J., Morishita, L., & Reed, R. (1995). Case management of older adults in health maintenance organizations. *Journal of the American Geriatric Society, 43,* 538–542.

Pacala, J., Boult, C., Reed, R., & Aliberti, E. (1997). Predictive validity of the Pra instrument among older recipients of managed care [see comments]. *Journal of the American Geriatrics Society, 45,* 614–617.

Parker, C. (1995). Practice guidelines and private insurers. *Journal of Law, Medicine and Ethics, 23,* 57–61.
Pauly, M. (1995). Practice guidelines: Can they save money? Should they? *Journal of Law, Medicine and Ethics, 23,* 65–74.
Polich, C., Bayard, J., Jacobson, R., & Parker, M. (1990). A nurse-run business to improve health care for nursing home residents. *Nursing Economics, 8,* 96–101.
Preston, J., & Retchin, S. (1991). The management of geriatric hypertension in health maintenance organizations. *Journal of the American Geriatric Society, 39,* 683–690.
Ramsey, S., & Pauly, M. (1997). Structural incentives and adoption of medical technologies in HMO and fee-for-service health insurance plans. *Inquiry, 34,* 228–236.
Remler, D., Donelan, K., Blendon, R., Lundberg, G., Leape, L., Calkins, D., Binns, K., & Newhouse, J. (1997). What do managed care plans do to affect care? Results from a survey of physicians. *Inquiry, 34,* 196–204.
Retchin, S., & Brown, B. (1990b). Quality of ambulatory care in Medicare health maintenance organizations. *American Journal of Public Health, 80,* 411–415.
Retchin, S., & Brown, B. (1990a). Management of colorectal cancer in Medicare health maintenance organizations. *Journal of General Internal Medicine, 5,* 110–114.
Retchin, S., & Brown, B. (1991). Elderly patients with congestive heart failure under prepaid care. *American Journal of Medicine, 90,* 236–242.
Retchin, S., Clement, D., & Brown, R. (1994). Care of patients hospitalized with strokes under the Medicare risk program. In H. Luft (Ed.), *HMOs and the elderly* (pp. 167–194). Ann Arbor, MI: Health Administration Press.
Retchin, S., & Preston, J. (1991). The effects of cost containment on the care of elderly diabetics. *Archives of Internal Medicine, 151,* 2244–2248.
Riley, G., Tudor, C., Chiang, Y., & Ingber, M. (1996). Health Status of Medicare enrollees in HMOs and fee-for-service in 1994. *Health Care Financing Review, 17,* 65–76.
Rossiter, L., Langwell, K., Wang, T., & Rivnyak, M. (1989). Patient satisfaction among elderly enrollees and disenrollees in Medicare Health Maintenance Organizations. *Journal of the American Medical Association, 262,* 57–63.
Rubenstein, L., Kahn, K., Reinisch, E., Sherwood, M., Rogers, W., Kamberg, C., Draper, D., & Brook, R. (1990). Changes in quality of care for five diseases measured by implicit review, 1981 to 1986. *Journal of the American Medical Society, 264,* 1974–1979.
Shaughnessy, P., Schlenker, R., & Hittle, D. (1994). Home health care outcomes under capitated and fee-for-service payment. *Health Care Financing Review, 16,* 187–221.
Tunis, S., Hayward, R., Wilson, M., Rubin, H., Bass, E., Johnston, M., & Steinberg, E. (1994). Internists' attitudes about clinical practice guidelines. *Annals of Internal Medicine, 120,* 956–963.
Wagner, E. (1997). Managed care and chronic illness. *Health Services Research, 32,* 702–714.

Ware, J., Bayliss, M., Rogers, W., Kosinski, M., & Tarlov, A. (1996). Differences in 4-year health outcomes for elderly and poor, chronically ill patients treated in HMO and fee-for-service systems. *Journal of the American Medical Association, 276*, 1039–1047.

Zarabozo, C., Taylor, C., & Hicks, J. (1996). Medicare managed care: Numbers and trends. *Health Care Financing Review, 17*, 243–261.

7
The "Voluntary" Status of Nursing Facility Admissions: Legal, Practice, and Public Policy Implications

Marshall B. Kapp

BACKGROUND

The Problem

In every jurisdiction within the United States, statutes permit the state to involuntarily hospitalize in a public mental health institution—or in a private institution that has been licensed by the state for this purpose—those persons who, because of mental illness, are considered dangerous to themselves or others (Appelbaum, 1994). By contrast, every admission of a new resident to a nursing facility, defined at 42 Code of Federal Regulations §440.155(a), (whether public, proprietary, or private not-for-profit) is, in theory, voluntary. Legal authority to involuntarily commit an individual to a nursing facility does not exist. Put differently, the law presumes that every admission to a nursing facility (like every other

---

Note: This article was published previously in the *New England Journal on Criminal and Civil Confinement*, Volume 24, No. 1. Reprinted with permission.

health care decision) (Faden & Beauchamp, 1986) is based, not only on a physician's order (Ouslander & Osterweil, 1994), but also on the informed, competent, and voluntary agreement (Kisor, 1996) either of the new resident personally or that of a legally authorized surrogate decision maker.

For instance, many nursing facility admissions result directly from hospital discharge planning processes. Federal Medicare regulations pertaining to these processes require that the hospital "must discuss the results of the [patient's discharge planning] evaluation with the patient or individual acting on his or her behalf" (42 Code of Federal Regulations §482.43(b)(6)). Other routes to a nursing facility include the hospital emergency department and the individual's home, particularly in situations where, shortly after hospital discharge, the individual and/or family finds that they are unable to cope adequately with the demands of home care. In each of these situations, voluntary informed consent to nursing facility admission is presumed as a matter of law.

In reality, many individuals have been "voluntarily" (Brooke, 1991–1992) admitted to nursing facilities even though

> (1) the resident personally lacks sufficient mental capacity to engage in a rational decisionmaking process (Smyer, Schaie, & Kapp, 1995) but has not been formally adjudicated incompetent by the local court of appropriate jurisdiction, and either
> (2) no interested family members (Brock, 1996) are available at the time of admission or
> (3) interested family members are available but have not been formally authorized to act as surrogate decision makers through a guardianship/conservatorship order or a previously executed durable power of attorney instrument.

In these situations, as a matter of practicality, nursing facilities ordinarily have accepted de facto decisionally incapacitated new residents despite the legal ambiguity surrounding their admission, and negative legal consequences to the nursing facility for proceeding in this manner have not materialized (Barton, Millik, Orr, & Janofsky, 1996).

However, widespread anecdotal reports, primarily from hospital discharge planners and geriatric care managers, indicate an increasing reluctance and in some cases unwillingness on the part of many nursing facility admission directors to continue to engage in these kinds of admissions on a routine basis. There is concern about current federal laws, mainly the Nursing Home Quality Reform Act included in the Omnibus Budget Reconciliation Act of 1987, 42 United States Code §§1395r-i(3)(a)-(h) (Medicare) and 1396r(a)-(h) (Medicaid) (Elon & Pawlson, 1992) and implementing regulations, 42 Code of Federal Regulations §483.10, and the Patient Self-Determination Act (PSDA) of 1990, 42 United States Code §§1395cc, 1396a), as well as about state laws and the government surveyors who enforce them. These laws and enforcers place strong emphasis upon resident autonomy (exercised either directly or through a surrogate), 42 Code of Federal Regulations §483.10(B)(4), in decision making within nursing facilities. This emphasis fosters apprehension by facilities about possible regulatory sanctions and/or civil liability for violating residents' autonomy (Kapp, 1995a; Kazin, 1989). Many nursing facility admission directors increasingly appear to be balking at accepting new residents on a "voluntary" admission status unless either the present decisional capacity of the resident or explicit legal authority on the part of the putative surrogate is clearly established and documented.

Greatest difficulty in effectuating nursing facility or other long-term care placement occurs in the case of severely psychotic individuals with significant behavioral problems and no visible surrogates, since facilities are concerned about their legal authority to, if necessary, physically restrain and/or treat such individuals with psychotropic drugs that carry substantial risks. Nursing facilities are prohibited by Title III of the Americans With Disabilities Act (ADA), 42 United States Code §§12181-12189 (Gottlich, 1994) and the Rehabilitation Act of 1973, 29 United States Code §794, from discriminating in admissions on the basis of an applicant's handicap, but they can deny admission to persons exhibiting dangerously aggressive behavior that the particular facility is not equipped to handle and care for properly (*Wagner*, 1995). Payment source also still often affects one's likelihood of being admitted to the nursing facility of his or her choice, as discrimination against Medicaid-eligible individuals still persists to a degree (Reschovsky, 1996) despite its current illegality in most states (Gilbert, 1991). Nursing facilities are under great pressure not to err in admitting individuals who will pose significant management problems, since it is extremely difficult legally to transfer or discharge a resident over objection once admission has occurred, 42 Code of Federal Regulations §483.12(a)(2) (Knepper, 1996).

In light of nursing facility reluctance to admit certain types of individuals, some discharge planners and care managers complain that a number of persons who should be transferred to nursing facilities from hospitals (who are not allowed to abandon these persons (Conrad, 1992)) or unsafe home environments are having those transfers delayed or disrupted until the legal question of who may voluntarily consent to the nursing facility admission is clarified. Such delays often work to the physical and emotional detriment of the eventual resident as well as the financial detriment of the hospital, and the resulting "solution" is frequently the initiation and imposition of a guardianship on the individual.

The legal and ethical literature fairly teems with discussions of personal autonomy in the context of treatment and daily living decisions to be made by individuals once they have become nursing facility residents (McCullough & Wilson, 1995). However, the informed consent status of nursing facility admissions in the first place has thus far been virtually ignored by legal practitioners, lawmakers, and scholars. For example, the extensive federal regulations and state statutes on residents' rights are totally silent on the admissions status issue. Current literature consists of a very few tangential allusions to the issue dealing mainly with ethical rather than legal considerations (Moody, 1987).

Potential Constitutional Considerations

A complicating factor in dealing with the status of nursing facility admissions is the potential impact of the United States Supreme Court's decision in the case of *Zinermon* v. *Burch* (1990) (Appelbaum, 1990). There, the Court ruled that the state of Florida could be sued civilly for permitting an adult person (who was later held to be mentally incompetent) to "voluntarily" admit himself to a public mental institution without first explicitly ascertaining and documenting that the patient possessed sufficient cognitive and emotional capacity to make an autonomous decision about his admission.

Although the *Zinermon* reasoning has not been applied yet to the nursing facility context, either in any litigated cases or the legal literature, the potential for such an application and its probable consequences must be considered. Admission practices of public facilities clearly implicate the "state action" that is necessary to trigger constitutional protections for the resident, and the extensive regulatory and financing (i.e., Medicare and Medicaid) entanglements between privately owned nursing facilities and government may be sufficient to satisfy the "state action" criterion for them as well (Thomas, 1982).

The Admissions Issue in Larger Perspective

The legal status of nursing facility admissions in the absence of a decisionally capable resident or a legally authorized surrogate is just one part of a larger situation concerning medical and other decision making for *de facto* incapable persons who are without families or close friends (Kapp,

1995b; Meier, 1997; Miller, Coleman, & Cugliari, 1997). The problem also arises, for instance, once a nursing facility resident who is or who becomes severely cognitively and/or emotionally impaired (and most nursing facility residents fall into this category (Burns et al., 1993)) needs specific interventions in the facility (e.g., restraints or particularly risky and invasive medications and medical procedures) and there is no clearly authorized surrogate willing and available to act.

Similarly, nursing facility residents often need to be transferred to acute care hospitals for treatment of specific problems, and the hospital (that is, the hospital's physicians, from whom all admitting and treatment orders must derive) may refuse to accept a person from the nursing facility and/or treat him or her in the absence of explicit legal authority. In extreme cases cited by nursing facility social service personnel, hospitals may refuse to dispose of a deceased patient's body until the transferring nursing facility administrator requests, albeit without any legal authority to do so, that the body be taken to a funeral home.

Additionally, hospital discharge planners may encounter difficulty in finding home health agencies that will accept "unbefriended" patients of questionable decisional capacity, particularly when the patient is requesting discharge to a physically risky home setting. These other types of situations are difficult and sorely in need of expeditious public policy attention, but their resolution is beyond the scope of the current report, which concentrates on the challenges of nursing facility admissions for the incapacitated unbefriended.

METHODS

Information Sources

To explore the legal, practice, and public policy issues raised in the preceding section, the author engaged in a qualitative research project from late 1996 through early 1997. In addition to an extensive review of the relevant literature (albeit with limited productivity), primary legal sources, and selected secondary materials, the research consisted of 30 structured interviews conducted by the author, either in person or by telephone, with five hospital discharge planners (chosen as a matter of convenience from hospitals of various sizes in southwestern Ohio); five nursing facility admissions personnel (chosen as a matter of convenience from facilities of various sizes and ownership statuses in southwestern Ohio); the state long-term care ombudsman and eight local long-term care ombudsmen from throughout Ohio, based on who responded favorably to a letter of inquiry sent to every local LTC ombudsman in the state); regulatory officials in the state health and aging departments; and leadership staff with the two chief nursing facility trade associations in Ohio, as well as representatives of the two major national nursing facility trade associations and seven consumer advocacy organizations. This report presents the author's observations and reflections founded on these sources of data and on less formal conversations with numerous other individuals about these issues. Statements presented in quotation marks are direct quotes from interviewees.

The survey methodology just described entails some obvious shortcomings. The number of interviews conducted was limited, as was the geographic area from which interviewees came. Convenience was one important selection criterion. Nonetheless, the fact that most persons interviewed answered the same questions posed in a quite similar manner, coupled with verification of these answers by nursing facility trade association officials and consumer advocates with a national perspective, provides good indication that the results of this survey are highly generalizable. While no attempt has been made here to precisely quantify the problem or extend the survey methodology beyond its present pilot status, data from all sources tapped appear to point uniformly in the direction of a significant set of concerns on the national level.

Research Questions

The major research questions posed during the structured xinterviews were:

- Are nursing facility admission directors reluctant to accept new residents unless the resident or a surrogate has clear legal authority to voluntarily consent to admission? If so, to what extent and how does this reluctance influence actual nursing facility practices?
- To the extent that a problem exists, how do hospital discharge planners deal with it? If there are delays in the transfer of individuals from the hospital to a suitable nursing facility, how do these delays affect the various actors medically, financially, and legally?
- In practice, how are evaluations made concerning the decisionmaking capacity of individuals seeking admission to nursing facilities? What process is followed, and who makes these decisions? What substantive standards are used for this evaluation?

- To the extent that legal uncertainty about the voluntariness issue exacerbates risk apprehension among nursing facilities and hospitals, and this apprehension is reflected in changed practice, has there been a significant impact on the number of guardianships initiated and awarded solely or primarily to authorize someone specific who can legally voluntarily consent to nursing facility admission for decisionally incapacitated persons? If so, who actually initiates and pays for these extra guardianship proceedings, and who becomes the guardian? Is the result unnecessary and/or premature guardianships, thus counteracting the autonomy-enhancing intent of current residents' rights laws? (Iris, 1990; Lisi, Burns, & Lussenden, 1994).
- To the extent that nursing facilities' legal apprehensions bring about socially undesirable outcomes regarding the care and placement of vulnerable individuals, what educational, public policy, and other types of interventions might be appropriate to address this problem?

FINDINGS

Legal Anxieties and Practice Implications

Most of the participants from nursing facilities expressed anxiety about the legality of admitting individuals for whom legal decisionmaking status is not clearly delineated, i.e., persons who are de facto seriously cognitively and/or emotionally impaired but who have not been adjudicated incompetent and who have no willing, available family members or friends to act as surrogate decision maker ("unbefriended" persons). When *any* willing and available family member (of any degree of relationship) or friend can be located, almost invariably facilities automatically accept that person as surrogate decision maker for the resident with no specific inquiry into the source, if any (and usually there is none), of that person's formal authority. This practice is not enshrined in written protocols but is virtually universally relied upon among long-term care professionals.

Without such a "warm body" with at least sufficient decisionmaking capacity (defined by one admissions officer interviewed for this project as the ability "to put an X on a piece of paper"), contemporary nursing facilities harbor anxieties that stem from uncertainty—not just about the legal validity of the admission itself, but also about future legal difficulties in obtaining payment (including getting Medicaid eligibility applications filed timely and correctly and on time); handling other financial matters; and obtaining consent for the initiation (e.g., transfers to acute facilities for emergency treatment) or discontinuation (e.g., removal of a ventilator or artificial feeding tubes) of specific medical interventions for the resident in legal limbo. Today's surrogates may drop out of the picture tomorrow, as they die, become incapacitated themselves, or decide that the needs of an increasingly aging, demented resident exceed their own abilities and tolerance for stress. Some nursing facilities still use blanket written consent-to-treatment forms at the time of admission, but that practice just raises the stakes of properly clarifying the resident's decisional capacity and/or the surrogate's authority at that early point in time.

Respondents reported that in the past, nursing facilities ordinarily were willing to act informally in the best interests of incapacitated unbefriended individuals, but they tend to be considerably more sensitive now about perceived liability considerations. Between federal OBRA provisions requiring that there be an indication on the resident's chart of the designated person to contact regarding the exercise of that person's rights; publicity about the PSDA and advance directives generally (King, 1996); anxieties that regulatory agency surveyors will act inconsistently and unpredictably; and the omnipresent exaggerated (Kapp, 1997; Meisel, 1995) but sincere fear of the "daughter from California" (Molloy, Clarnette, Braun, Eisemann, & Sneiderman, 1991) who will suddenly show up and complain at the last instant that "Dad shouldn't have been allowed to wander," many nursing facility administrators describe themselves as being "paranoid" about their exposure to potential liability for doing anything to a person without clear delineation of who has the legal authority to provide valid informed consent or refusal of services. This feeling is especially intense when the potential resident, even if not mentally capable to make such a decision, is manifesting an active objection to institutional placement.

Although most administrators and their staffs intellectually understand that regulatory and/or civil liability repercussions in this area are rare, these repercussions (or, just as importantly, the threat of them) are a very disruptive, time- and resource-intensive "big deal" when they do materialize. Several nursing facility interviewees reported being initially cited by state surveyors for failing to have a specific surrogate identified in a resident's chart, and being instructed "simplistically" by the survey team to "just find somebody for this guy." The nursing facilities' pervasive feeling of uneasiness is exacerbated, according to one ombudsman interviewee, by the negative reaction of more than a few probate judges, who react less than pleasantly to being bothered in the middle of the night with a request for emergency authorization to do something to, or for, a resident who lacks both decisional capacity and relatives.

Nursing facilities are most apprehensive about admitting seriously psychotic, demented, or developmentally disabled persons with violent, aggressive behavioral problems. In addition to concerns about their ability to care properly for such individuals in light of available staffing and physical plant limitations, there is apprehension by facilities about the anticipated potential future need for someone to validly consent (over the resident's objection, if necessary) to the use of physical restraints, psychotropic medications, and/or transfer to a more secure facility, as well as concern about the handling of payment and other financial matters.

According to several nursing facility admissions officers interviewed for this project, nursing facilities' insistence on clear identification of a surrogate decision maker prior to admitting a new resident who is expected to present behavioral problems is driven, at least in part, by experiences with hospital psychiatry units that "refuse to accept" resident transfers unless a surrogate has been named in a durable power of attorney instrument (Frolik & Brown, 1992) or through a guardianship order (Frolik & Kaplan, 1995). In this realm, the admissions policies of many nursing facilities and hospitals may be legally questionable, in light of the PSDA's explicit prohibition against requiring the execution of an advance directive as a precondition to a patient/resident's admission, Public Law No. 101-508, §§4206(f)(1)(C) and 4751(2)(C).

Persons interviewed for this project also noted that transfers of incapacitated unbefriended individuals from their own homes to a nursing facility usually were more difficult to effectuate than hospital-to-nursing facility transfers. Reasons for this include nursing facilities' concerns about PASARR (Preadmission Screening and Resident Review Assessment) screenings—which may result in Medicaid refusing to pay for nursing facility care of an individual who is determined to have a primary mental illness diagnosis—and getting Medicaid eligibility applications completed in a timely fashion. In some communities, physicians on the local hospital's medical staff sometimes ask the hospital's social service personnel for assistance in satisfying those details on behalf of community-dwelling patients who need nursing facility admittance.

Financial Influences

Interestingly, how widespread legal skittishness on the nursing facilities' part actually gets translated into admissions practice appears to vary greatly, depending on how occupied a particular facility happens to be on a given day, i.e., how competitive a facility needs to be in order to fill its revenue-producing beds. Legal fears may often be expressed, to a certain degree at least, as a pretext for financial considerations. "Adaptability," according to one hospital social service director, "is a function of present census" and the availability of someone who is willing and able to sign an admissions contract and/or Medicaid application (and to grant access to the applicant's financial records so that financial eligibility for this means-tested program can be verified) that guarantees payment. In the final analysis, "Admissions are a business decision" and "We are not Moms and Pops any more."

In Ohio in 1996, total nursing facility occupancy stood at 91.8%, with substantial variation among specific facilities. Largely as a result of the success of federal requirements for pre-screening potential residents for mental health and retardation problems, 42 Code of Federal Regulations Part 483, Subpart C, state home and community-based Medicaid waiver initiatives such as Ohio's PASSPORT program, Ohio Revised Code §5101.75 *et. seq.*, and prospective utilization review requirements of private long-term care insurance policies, more older people with substantial deficiencies in performing activities of daily living (ADLs) (i.e., bathing, dressing, getting in or out of bed or chair, toileting, and eating) are able today to reside outside of nursing facilities, and few get admitted unnecessarily or prematurely, at least directly from the community. (The problem of physicians and managed care case managers too readily recommending nursing facility placement following an older individual's hospitalization is discussed in the Implications section, below.)

The upshot of these factors, coupled with loosened certificate-of-need requirements and easy access to venture capital leading to more building of nursing facilities, assisted living, and subacute entities, is that additional beds have been built and the nursing facility industry has become increasingly competitive in recent years. One of the primary customers to be cultivated in such a competitive environment is the hospital discharge planner who substantially influences the flow of post-hospital consumers and the dollars that follow them. Discharge planners, in turn, have a symbiotic relationship with nursing facility admissions officers; these professionals need, and hence have a strong incentive, to work positively with each other. All in all, the growing competitive climate may ease difficulties in placing now hard-to-place individuals in need of long-term care.

Already, facilities with a significant number of beds to fill often manage to "overcome" their apprehensions about the legal status of applicants for admission much more readily than do those who enjoy the current luxury of waiting lists. Facilities in the former category tend to employ a much looser working threshold for decisional capacity, relying more readily on the applicant's own signature during a "lucid" moment, than do their fully occupied counterparts (although the latter claim to continue to worry and ask questions about the legal ramifications of the residents they have admitted in this condition).

Thus, according to several project interviewees, the most dependent and vulnerable individuals, sometimes as a last resort, are placed in nursing facilities of the most dubious quality, since such providers are the most likely to temper their concerns about an unbefriended individual's legal status—and their own capacity to properly care for that individual—in order to fill, and pay for, their beds. They are "most willing not to stand on technicalities," according to one ombudsman, when the individual has already been certified eligible for Medicaid or has another definitive source of financial coverage for services. The "most hungry" nursing facilities may even initiate the Medicaid application process for a new resident, a burden that other facilities firmly insist should be shouldered by hospital social service departments or community case managers.

These "hungry" facilities are well-known to hospital discharge planners who, although frequently uncomfortable with these placements, can take solace in the fact that ultimately "every applicant gets in somewhere." For especially undesirable unbefriended persons, such as older individuals with alcohol-related dementia and associated behavioral problems, there may be a need to rely on specialized facilities in distant locations for placement.

Conversely, many of the best local facilities can afford to be the most selective regarding admissions, and therefore act the most conservatively in restricting access to their services to persons of more certain legal status (i.e., not accepting applicants who lack an available family member or friend to act as present or future surrogate). The most conservative facilities (i.e., usually those with the longest waiting lists) may go so far as to illegally require a third party to sign the admissions contract even if the applicant is not mentally impaired, in a tactic to avoid future management problems.

Several consumer advocates interviewed for this project noted, with a touch of skepticism, that when nursing facilities resist admitting an individual without a specific surrogate decision maker already in place, they publicly justify their conduct on grounds of residents' rights (and "company policy"), rather than as a concern about their own liability risk, or the fact that they simply prefer not to admit particular categories of persons who are likely to command an inordinate amount of work and attention. As one nursing facility admissions director admitted to the author, it is "just easier" for the facility to deal with situations when there is an identified surrogate. "That way, we know the paperwork will be done."

A slight variation on the picture described above may be found in the case of some comprehensive continuing care retirement communities offering multiple levels of care. In that setting, when a person living in a community's independent or assisted living sections develops an acute medical problem necessitating hospital admission followed by transfer to nursing facility-level care, that community's nursing facility may be willing to accept the person (who is already known to the staff) despite a legally uncertain status and a healthy institutional census. Even in this situation, though, the nursing facility ordinarily will initiate an immediate attempt (see guardianship discussion, below) to formally clarify legal decisionmaking authority for that resident.

Impact on the Parties

The practices described above exert a tangible, direct impact on the various parties. For the older individual in need of timely nursing facility placement, delays of days or even weeks—and in a small number of extreme cases, months—have been reported, not as a regular matter but frequently enough to be notable. During these delays, the individual not only fails to receive appropriate nursing facility care, but is unnecessarily exposed to potential infections and the other risks attendant to the hospital inpatient setting. Since these unduly extended hospitalizations ordinarily are grossly inadequately compensated under Medicare's prospective payment system of Diagnosis Related Groups (DRGs), 42 Code of Federal Regulations Part 412, the financial repercussions for a hospital (and there is wide variation among hospitals in this regard) may be dire.

Understandably, the hospital always has strong financial, ethical, and clinical incentives to expedite appropriate placement of individuals outside of the hospital. One hospital social service director told the author about the 1995 patient whose unnecessarily extended stay cost her hospital over $100,000 because no one had legal authority to sell the property that made the patient ineligible for Medicaid and therefore unable to be placed in a nursing facility; numerous versions of this anecdote were repeated in hospitals across Ohio. Most hospitals today possess a computer system that tracks medically "avoidable patient days," as well as the department (e.g., Social Services) that is responsible for those money-losing days, thereby precisely focusing pressure to move the patient out.

Financial considerations aside, there are other factors driving hospitals, as well as nursing facilities, to seek legally definitive resolutions to decisionmaking quandaries involving mentally impaired, unbefriended persons. When there is doubt about the individual's decisional capacity and/

or the safety of the treatment plan, there often is a great temptation for hospital staff to circumvent the moral dilemmas by "letting the judge decide." Defensive medicine considerations also may come into play; the hospital that fears potential civil liability for injuries suffered by a de facto incapacitated but unadjudicated person whom it improperly sends home to an unsafe environment has a reason to seek guardianship, so that the individual can be placed in what is believed to be a more secure, protective nursing facility setting.

Nursing facilities must deal chiefly with their apprehensiveness about potential regulatory liability. If state surveyors find that the provision of proper care for a mentally incapacitated nursing facility resident has been hampered by the absence of a guardian or other legally authorized decision maker, the regulatory agency likely will require the nursing facility to move toward obtaining guardianship in order to obtain informed consent to the care that has previously been withheld. Some consumer advocates related to the author their personal observations (or those of volunteer guardians or long-term care ombudsmen) of nursing facility residents who had been denied desirable elective medical treatments (e.g., corrective cataract surgery, hernia repair) because there was no legally authorized surrogate decision maker to give valid consent to these quality-of-life enhancing interventions. The expectation that surveyors are unlikely to exert pressure toward guardianship, as long as it appears that the quality of care being rendered to an incapacitated resident is acceptable, provides only limited comfort to most nursing facilities, especially in the absence of official, practical guidance in this regard emanating from government agencies.

Current Strategies

In response to the financial, legal, and other incentives enumerated, most hospitals have devised (although often reluctantly) systems for initiating guardianships for mentally impaired, unbefriended patients for whom the only obstacle to needed nursing facility placement is the absence of a legally authorized surrogate decision maker. Operating such a system may entail a substantial financial commitment on the hospital's part, but it is ordinarily extremely cost-effective, as compared with the potential losses to which a hospital is exposed as a result of unnecessarily extended, prospectively priced inpatient hospital stays for the individuals for whom nursing facility placement would otherwise be delayed.

The various surrogate-delineation systems currently found in the context of incapacitated unbefriended persons needing nursing facility placement vary in several important details. These particulars include:

- Who actually initiates the guardianship, and who acts as the guardian?
- Who pays for the processing of the guardianship petition, and who pays for the conduct of the guardianship itself?
- What is the extent of the guardian's authority?

In one common model, the hospital files the guardianship petition (often initially on an emergency basis, Ohio Revised Code §2111.02, and later for an indefinite order); provides and pays the professional team consisting of a psychiatrist, psychologist, and social worker to evaluate the individual's decisional capacity, submit its report to the court, and testify if necessary; and hires a private attorney to serve as guardian. Usually, the retained attorney accepts authority over financial matters, while procuring and paying for (on behalf of the hospital) a nonprofit or proprietary social service agency for the court to appoint as guardian of the person. In return for the efficiency achieved in transferring the individual to a nursing facility, the hospital bears associated expenses (unless the individual involved has sufficient assets from which the guardian may be paid by court order) and is exposed to possible charges of at the least an appearance of conflict of interest.

In another model, hospitals—as well as home health agencies, Area Agencies on Aging, case managers, and others concerned with the proper placement of the unbefriended individual—work with volunteer guardianship programs in the initiation and conduct of a judicially appointed surrogate decisionmaking arrangement. Volunteer guardianship programs have been established by a variety of charitable entities (often religiously or civicly affiliated) to have someone who is willing and able to be appointed as an incapacitated person's surrogate decision maker when there is no other suitable candidate (Fins, 1992; Gibson & Nathanson, 1990; Zimny & Diamond, 1994).

In Ohio, volunteer guardianship programs presently operate in, among a number of other places, Montgomery, Franklin, Richland, and Cuyahoga counties. These programs are funded from a variety of sources, such as the local hospital association (e.g., Montgomery County's CHUMS program is funded in major part by the Greater Dayton Area Hospital Association, entailing an obvious seeming conflict of interest), Area Agencies on Aging, county indigent guardianship funds, Ohio Revised Code §2111.51, funds generated by litigation filing fees or interest on attorneys' trust accounts, United Way allocations, contributions by religious congregations and civic groups, private donations, and grants.

Several states have legislatively created public guardianship systems in which government agencies, or private agencies under contract or other arrangement with the government, at the state or local level are available for court appointment as the decisionmaking agent of last resort for the unbefriended in need of formal surrogacy. For example, in Maryland the director of the state or local office on aging may be appointed guardian in such situations.

Many of these systems are limited and specialized. In Ohio, for example, public guardianship is available only for children and decisionally incapacitated developmentally disabled adults, but not for adults who are severely cognitively and/or emotionally impaired due to dementia, depression, psychosis, or other reason than developmental disability.

In the absence of one of the kinds of arrangements outlined above, it may be exceedingly difficult to accomplish a guardianship for a mentally impaired, unbefriended elder in need of nursing facility placement. Attorneys are reluctant to agree to provide their services in the absence of assurance that their time will be compensated reasonably. Private, proprietary guardianship corporations make themselves unavailable for appointment when an individual's estate lacks sufficient assets to pay their fees. Private individuals, such as social friends, religious pastors and fellow congregants, and the like, may be intimidated—and thus unwilling to accept guardianship—by the perceived onerous responsibilities of difficult personal and financial decision making for an increasingly demented, often impoverished individual over what could be a lengthy period of time. Additionally, infrequent but invariably well-publicized scandals about misuse of funds or abuse of a ward by a guardian always exert a discouraging impact on potential guardian recruitment in the scandal's locality.

Accurate national figures describing the extent and nature of contemporary guardianship are difficult to obtain (Schmidt, 1995). There was a broad, but not quite unanimous, consensus among the professionals interviewed for this project that today the number of inappropriate or premature guardianships imposed involuntarily on older persons is relatively small. Put differently, the vast majority of interviewees maintained that guardianship for mentally incapacitated unbefriended individuals is sought overwhelmingly only as a last resort.

Hospitals initiate a significant number of guardianships, preliminary to nursing facility placement, directly from emergency departments (where some of the larger hospitals now assign full-time social workers for this purpose). Many of these cases involve scenarios where a family needs the individual's Social Security retirement check and therefore keeps caring for the person inadequately at home, bringing her to the emergency department for specific problems, taking her home again, and then repeating the cycle until the hospital feels ethically compelled to intervene. Such intervention is most likely when the emergency squad has brought the individual into the hospital emergency department and provided the social service department with a "social concerns" report on the individual's atrocious living conditions.

The precipitating event for the pursuit of a guardianship petition usually is a specific, immediate need of a third party (e.g., a health care provider and/or financial institution) for legal clarification of legitimate decision-making authority. An attempt by a dementia unit resident to sign himself out of a nursing facility, thereby worrying the facility about its own possible legal exposure, is a prime example of such an event.

Otherwise, especially for indigent persons who have no resources to support surrogate decisionmaking services (Whitton, 1996), decision making for the incapacitated unbefriended tends to be a haphazardly jerry-built type of affair. Muddling through on an ad hoc basis may be characterized by reliance on the emergency exception to informed consent to eventually justify medical intervention (Richards & Rathbun, 1993), and important decisions dangerously deferred, foregone altogether, or conversely, defaulted to a maximum medical intervention position. Another alternative often observed is health care and human service providers acting either unilaterally or in combination as de facto surrogates but often covertly and with hesitation.

Issues of Decision-making Capacity

All of these approaches to surrogate decision making are based, of course, on the premise that a particular individual needs a surrogate because of personal incapacity in the first place. How nursing facility admissions personnel, hospital discharge planners, case managers, and even consumer advocates make this initial determination, prior to initiation of a guardianship petition or other surrogate arrangement for an unbefriended nursing facility candidate, appears to be a totally unstructured and unstandardized, ad hoc exercise, varying markedly among different nursing facilities and even different staff members within the same nursing facility, and from one candidate for nursing facility admission to another.

The picture of capacity assessment for voluntary admission purposes that emerged from this project's interviews is consistent with that portrayed in a recent study that examined assessment of capacity to participate in discussions of advance medical directives in nursing facilities. That study found that:

> When nursing home staff were probed about how they determine whether residents have the decision-making capacity to discuss advance directives and make end-of-life treatment choices, no clear process or procedure was

described; rather a variety of techniques were used to determine residents' capacity to discuss advance directives. . . . [T]here was no . . . explicit standard, and the judgment is left to the admissions staff. . . . In no case was there a formal policy and process of assessing cognitive ability or decisional capacity. Instead, the process of assessing residents' capacity . . . is nonstandard and often left to staff who have little procedural guidance from either institutional policy or the legal system (Bradley, Walker, Blechner, & Wetle, 1997).

Adult Protective Services

Persons interviewed for this project were ambivalent about the role of Adult Protective Services (APS), Ohio Revised Code §5101.60, in the context of nursing facility admissions for the incapacitated unbefriended. Many felt that the APS agencies' potential helpfulness is severely limited by a number of factors. First, insufficient resources lead to excessive burden on caseworkers. Second is the fact that persons who are already nursing facility residents are beyond the jurisdiction of APS on the theory that they are in a protective environment (although APS in some counties will continue to pursue a guardianship for a hospitalized unbefriended individual when the petition was filed while the person was living in the community). Third, there is the widely shared reputation of many APS agencies for not following through on the submission and processing of Medicaid eligibility applications for unbefriended individuals whom they have signed into nursing facilities.

Some interviewees also accused certain APS agencies of too readily seeking guardianship and institutional placement without adequate exploration of less restrictive alternatives, although generalizations are hard to draw when each county's APS system functions independently. In fact, the lack of communication and coordinated policies and procedures among APS agencies was cited by many as a major weakness.

Public policy implications of guardianship and its several permutations and alternatives, as well as the process of decisional capacity evaluation, are discussed in the following section. Private initiatives for protecting the incapacitated unbefriended who are nursing facility candidates, without sacrificing their autonomy-based rights, are outlined as well.

POLICY IMPLICATIONS

Themes

The key public policy challenge in this arena is the need to achieve a reasonable balance between bureaucratic intermeddling that, while well-meaning, is both overly paternalistic and palpably counterproductive, on the one hand, and excessively and unrealistically insistent on the hypothetical autonomy rights of an extremely vulnerable population, on the other (Barnes, 1992). With neither true autonomy to empower them nor true beneficence to protect them, incapacitated unbefriended individuals quite literally live with the constant danger of falling between the cracks of our modern social, ethical, and legal systems. Those who are sufficiently impaired physically and/or mentally to require nursing facility care are at particular risk.

How the policy challenge will be addressed and a reasonable balance sought will depend in large measure on how we resolve two philosophical questions with very practical consequences.

(1) What is the essential character of the modern nursing facility: health provider, mental health provider, and/or residential, homelike abode? (Wetle, 1995–1996)

(2) Ought we to be guided mainly by a medical/therapeutic model, that emphasizes protection of the vulnerable, dependent individual against harm and maximization of that person's physical and mental well-being, or by a legal/rights model (Murphy, 1996) that emphasizes substantive and procedural due process safeguards against exploitation and abuse?

Alternatives

With these overarching themes in mind, we may outline the principal alternatives. Most prominently, government might encourage and facilitate the appointment of guardians to act as official, legally authorized decisionmaking surrogates for incapacitated unbefriended candidates for nursing facility admission. This approach could resolve clearly, in a timely—even arguably a preemptively and proactively—fashion the legal status of those nursing facility admissions, as well as the legal status of the various decisions made on the resident's behalf at that time and subsequently.

There are approximately 25,000 adult guardianship cases adjudicated in Ohio each year. Ohio Revised Code §2111.02, consistent with the least restrictive alternative (LRA) principle and the statutes of every other state (Kapp, 1994), permits courts to appoint guardians with limited or partial powers tailored specifically to the actual cognitive and/or emotional deficits of the ward; nonetheless, courts create virtually all guardianships as plenary or complete transfers of legal authority from the ward to the guardian. In the same vein, although empowered to appoint guardians on a temporary basis in situations when the ward may be expected to regain decisional capacity, probate courts tend to disfavor this option and to appoint permanent guardians instead; the burden then falls to the ward to seek subsequent guardianship termination at a later date.

On the one hand, without detracting at all from the desirability of more independent, holistic geriatric assessments of potential wards to inform the probate courts, the bulk of professionals interviewed for this project suggested that the overwhelming majority of current guardianships are necessary both for the welfare and protection of the nursing facility applicant/resident and to safeguard the risk management interests of the nursing facility and other service providers. Their key concern was the fate of nursing facility unbefriended candidates who ought to have guardians, but who are likely to suffer discrimination and mistreatment because of the difficulties in obtaining this needed source of protection. Typical was the comment of one long-term care ombudsman that, while her office will not accept appointment as guardian for a nursing facility resident (for conflict of interest reasons), it has moved in the past few years from a knee-jerk opposition to all guardianship petitions toward facilitating the accomplishment of guardianship orders (including the identification of appropriate persons to be appointed) when a resident really needs a surrogate and no better alternatives exist.

Although the following recommendations were not unanimously endorsed by participants in this project, and some urged considerable misgivings about them, the substantial majority of project interviewees advocated government actions that would encourage and facilitate more guardianships by, for example:

- Enhancing legislative funding of county indigent guardianship funds, Ohio Revised Code §2111.51, mainly to entice more private attorneys and others to be willing to serve as conscientious (i.e., not pro forma) guardians for incapacitated unbefriended persons—including potential and actual nursing facility residents—who lack substantial income and assets. The setting of a specific, express fee schedule for paying appointed attorneys using indigent guardianship funds, rather than relying on ad hoc payment decisions by each probate court, may be helpful in this regard;
- Streamlining and economizing the guardianship process ("forgetting the red tape"). The current expensive and cumbersome process, in addition to its other shortcomings, frightens away many low-income families of Medicaid-eligible persons, thus making those persons unbefriended. A more "user-friendly" guardianship process might

sustain more family involvement. Additionally, many nursing facilities complain that, while they will accept an applicant once a guardianship petition has been filed—on the almost always borne-out presumption that the petition will be granted eventually—"the process takes much too long";
- Empowering APS agencies to initiate selectively (i.e., not for purposes of "dumping" somebody troublesome) guardianships for individuals who are in a hospital or nursing facility;
- Instilling more uniformity among probate courts in dealing with these issues, instead of the current "independent, inconsistent fiefdom" topography (e.g., divergence in how indigent guardianship funds are handled, receptivity of court investigators to health care provider requests for assistance) prevailing among county probate courts, including more of a case management and oversight role for the probate courts (although the Summit County probate court convened a meeting in late 1996 precisely to advise health and human services providers *not* to continue calling the court investigator for help in managing the daily problems of the unbefriended);
- Encouraging greater use by the courts of limited or partial guardianship (currently, a significant percentage of all limited guardianships created in Ohio are awarded to APSI for developmentally disabled wards), as well as guardianship *ad litem*, Ohio Revised Code §2111.23, when formal surrogacy is necessary only for a specific decision or for several decisions bunched together within a short period of time, such as acute hospitalization in the midst of nursing facility residency; and
- Recognizing some sort of limited "good faith" exception to the usual informed consent requirements in the case of "obviously" incapacitated unbefriended nursing facility applicants and residents.

In Ohio, public guardianship systems have been legislatively created for children, Ohio Revised Code §§2151.353, .413, .414, and developmentally disabled adults, Ohio Revised Code §5123.55-59, only. In 1971, the Ohio legislature established procedures for nonprofit corporate guardianship of citizens of any age with developmental disabilities severe enough to impair decisionmaking capacity, as well as unique trusteeship/protectorship programs. The Association for Retarded Citizens was the driving force behind the enabling legislation, because parents were worried about what would happen to their developmentally disabled children after their own deaths. Presently, the state contracts the surrogacy function created by this legislation to Advocacy and Protective Services, Inc. (APSI).

Public policymakers, including the Department of Aging, should carefully study the developmental disabilities model, as well as public guardianship systems in other states, to determine what elements—if any—might be appropriate for application to the situation of incapacitated unbefriended elders in need of nursing facility admission. Special attention might be paid to the trusteeship/protectorship status as an intermediate step between plenary guardianship, on the one hand, and nihilistic neglect, on the other. Such a study, however, must keep in mind that the actual extent and effectiveness of public guardianship programs probably depends more heavily on the resources that a jurisdiction appropriates for its operation (generally grossly insufficient) than on the terms of the enabling legislation (Siemon, Balch, Hurme, & Sabatino, 1993). Additionally, any new system setting up a contractual relationship with a private agency to perform public guardianship functions should avoid APSI-like conflicts of interest by strictly separating the guardianship agency from direct oversight by its state funder and thereby maintaining a more appropriate arm's-length relationship.

Assuming that actions to encourage and facilitate private, volunteer, and/or public guardianships are successful, the natural result would be a greater proliferation of guardianship petitions and orders and, consequently, an even greater reluctance on the part of nursing facilities to admit incapacitated unbefriended applicants in the absence of an explicitly authorized legal surrogacy arrangement. An obvious policy issue is whether such a state of affairs is desirable, as opposed to promoting guardianship alternatives that might better promote the unbefriendeds' welfare without unduly compromising their autonomy. Sponsored research producing data about whether or not the risk of abuse, neglect, or exploitation of nursing facility residents is in any way tied (and if so, how) to the absence of formal guardians—or whether residents with families, friends, or no one are just as likely to be mistreated or ignored—would be informative in working through that policy question.

At least two states (namely, New York (Herr & Hopkins, 1994) and California, Health and Safety Code §1418.8) have created an official, but nonjudicial, alternative to guardianship for unbefriended persons with mental disabilities. The California statute creating an administrative mechanism for approving interventions in nursing facilities for decisionally incapacitated residents with no legally authorized surrogate has been upheld against constitutional attack (*Rains v. Belshe*, 1995).

Harvard University geriatrician Muriel R. Gillick has proposed the development and dissemination of a new In-House Surrogate System, utilizing relevant nursing facility staff to make decisions for incapacitated unbefriended residents (Gillick, 1995). There is no compelling reason that some version of this sort of administrative structure could not be employed for making initial decisions about admitting particular nursing facility applicants. Indeed, in an analogous area, attorney Bruce Winick (1994) has urged use of informal administrative methods, rather than adversarial judicial proceedings, to determine a person's capacity to voluntarily consent to psychiatric hospitalization. Gillick's proposal is guided by the medical/therapeutic model alluded to above, giving primacy to the ethical principle of beneficence (Pellegrino & Thomasma, 1988).

A leading national nursing facility consumer advocate whose thinking is driven by the legal/rights model, however, criticizes Gillick's administrative system proposal as too laden with real and apparent conflicts of interest, preferring instead a high degree of role differentiation for nursing facility staff (Freeman, 1995). This criticism, interestingly, was not unanimously shared by the long-term care ombudsmen interviewed by the author; particularly those serving rural areas, where "everybody has known everybody forever," thought that having nursing facility staff act as surrogate decision makers of last resort made "natural sense."

While many existing volunteer guardianship programs are laudable, probably it is unrealistic to expect sufficient development and funding of this sector to address adequately the burgeoning need. By definition, these programs have minimal paid staff and depend heavily on the time, generosity, and reliability of individual volunteers, factors that are finite and largely unpredictable in a population consisting of persons who tend to be older themselves. Individual volunteers come and go for a panoply of reasons. While participating in the program, they need to be continually educated, reeducated, and supervised—no insignificant task. The willingness and ability of volunteer guardians to "push the system where necessary" has been questioned, too.

Exacerbating the unavoidable instability of volunteer guardianship programs, in Ohio, other than in the special situations of children or developmentally disabled adults, probate judges may appoint only a real person (as opposed to an agency *qua* agency) as a guardian, Ohio Revised Code §2111.10. Thus, when an individual volunteer guardian in a volunteer guardianship program for any reason terminates his or her participation, the agency sponsoring the volunteer guardianship program may need to return to court seeking appointment of a new individual volunteer as guardian. Many volunteer guardianship programs have recommended (although some are opposed to the idea) that the probate courts be empowered to bring about appointment of the agency *qua* agency, so that the comings and goings of particular volunteers may be dealt with as an internal, administrative matter by the agency rather than necessitating an additional judicial proceeding.

Current public guardianship programs were criticized by a number of interviewees for policies rejecting involvement in the cases of unbefriended individuals who have any financial assets. In many cases, these disqualifying assets are too insubstantial to attract willing private guardians, with the upshot that the person with some, but not much, assets remains in a state of legal limbo.

Another possible public policy approach lies in efforts to better align the concept of advance medical planning to the needs of incapacitated, unbefriended, would-be nursing facility residents (Mezey, Mitty, Rappaport, & Ramsey, 1997). Much attention has been devoted to the use of proxy directives, primarily durable powers of attorney, as a less restrictive alternative to guardianship. These legal mechanisms allow a presently decisionally capable adult to name in advance a proxy or substitute person to act as decision maker in the future contingency that the principal or maker (the party delegating away the authority) subsequently becomes incapacitated.

The chief problem for the population discussed in this report is that its members have no willing, able persons to name as their future decisionmaking agents in a durable power of attorney document, or else the persons whom they named as their agents earlier while still capable have now become unavailable or unwilling by the time that the principals have become incapacitated and actually need surrogate decision making. According to one legal commentator, one way to obviate this difficulty would be for the state legislature to explicitly authorize currently capable adults to prospectively appoint nonprofit (i.e., charitable) organizations as their surrogate decision makers at the time of future decisional incapacity (Whitton, 1996). These organizations could either be general social service providers, or set up specifically for the purpose of acting as surrogate decision maker of last resort. This approach would avoid the time, expense, administrative hassle, and emotional turmoil of a formal guardianship proceeding; permit the affected individual to maintain some degree of personal autonomy; and promote beneficent treatment of the individual by, for example, providing a protective but efficient means of effectuating appropriate admissions to and treatment within nursing facilities for those who cannot speak on their own behalfs.

Since assessments of individuals' decisional capacity prior to initiation of formal guardianship proceedings are essentially ad hoc, unguided, and inconsistent, a number of interviewees called for a greater degree of legal and professional guidance for capacity evaluators. Standardization of capacity evaluations promise greater objectivity and reliability of results, although quantitative measurements cannot completely take the place of clinical judgment (Kapp & Mossman, 1996).

Given that much of the hyperdefensive activity practiced by nursing facilities stems from anxiety about possible regulatory liability and sanctions, many interviewees suggested much more concerted training and information dissemination initiatives for state nursing facility surveyors and other relevant regulators about OBRA; the PSDA; state residents' rights laws; surrogate decision making; and the informed consent doctrine generally. Desired outcomes of these government sponsored continuing educational activities would include greater consistency and predictability in enforcement of legal requirements, more honest and realistic proactive communication between regulators and nursing facilities on these points, and ultimately a zone of legal comfort within which nursing facilities will feel freer to develop and implement more creative approaches to the clinical and ethical needs of incapacitated unbefriended applicants and residents.

Nongovernmental Initiatives

In terms of nongovernmental initiatives to improve the situations of incapacitated unbefriended persons in need of nursing facility placement, none of the persons the author interviewed mentioned the potential role of institutional ethics committees (IECs) in helping nursing facilities grapple successfully with difficult admissions questions. Perhaps this is because involved professionals conceptualize this subject area solely as a matter of pragmatic risk management rather than as one entailing serious ethical and policy dilemmas. Such a reading of the issues is excessively narrow. Nursing facilities should be encouraged to explore the possible salutary contributions of IECs in terms of help with institutional policy formulation, individual case consultation (concurrent or retrospective), and education of the nursing facility staff and other constituencies, including families (Hoffmann, Boyle, & Levenson, 1995).

Many interviewees called for more communication and education among hospitals, nursing facilities, and home care agencies about their respective environments and constraints. To address what is widely perceived as a deficit of mutual appreciation and understanding, at least one Ohio long-term care ombudsman established in 1996 an enthusiastically received hospital/nursing facility working group to deal with behavioral problems, including those pertaining to resident admission, transfer, and discharge. Ombudsman offices can also provide an invaluable service by conducting in-service training on a host of nursing facility admission-related topics.

Almost all the persons interviewed proposed actions to better educate physicians about post-hospital care of the chronically disabled, including the incapacitated unbefriended patient population. While (as discussed earlier) most discharge planners, nursing facility admissions staff, and consumer advocates believe that programs to divert people from unnecessary institutionalization have been largely effective, these same parties charge that many physicians are poorly informed about these less restrictive long-term care alternatives and about level of care issues generally. Consequently, they lament, physicians on the whole are not very helpful in finessing the problems associated with nursing facility admissions for incapacitated unbefriended individuals; more formal training in this area is imperative.

Similarly, many interviewees observed that managed care case managers often have limited backgrounds regarding long-term care, and hence show a tendency to equate the entire field with nursing facilities. More education of this increasingly powerful profession about the range of long-term care settings and opportunities should be strongly encouraged.

More education was also endorsed for other service providers, particularly nursing facility administrators and staffs. Long-term care ombudsmen and other resident advocates cited significant deficiencies in accurate provider knowledge of the relevant law, often leading to either an ignoring of resident treatment wishes (i.e., "We're in doubt, so we better provide the full-court press") or an overinterpretation of advance directives or other apparent treatment refusals serving as an excuse to abandon troublesome residents rather than to personalize their care.

A comprehensive recommendation endorsed by all of the interviewees addresses the lack of consistency and predictability in practice and policy that was widely lamented. It calls for the creation of a process through which key actors concerned with the problems raised by nursing facility care for incapacitated unbefriended individuals could meaningfully communicate and discuss from their multiple perspectives the issues outlined in this report, with the goal of formulating and ultimately disseminating a set of broadly acceptable policies and procedures. In this way, a solid core of common expectations and uniform national approaches could be promulgated and promoted to service providers, regulators, and consumer advocates relating to the welfare and rights of this especially vulnerable and expanding group of persons. This collaborative, consensus building process could spring from both public and private (e.g., foundation) support.

CONCLUSION

The phenomenon of unbefriended, severely and chronically mentally incapacitated older individuals in need of nursing facility-level care can only continue to grow. As a result of increased life expectancy and other demographic trends, the elderly will constitute an increasing share of the American population as we move to the new millennium. By 2030, about one-fifth of our population will be at least 65 years old, compared with barely 13% currently, and less than 10% in 1970. The proportion of the population age 85 and older is expected to rise from 1.4% in 1996 to 2% in 2010 and to almost 5% by 2050 (Komisar, Lambrew, & Feder, 1996, p. 72).

A portion of this group will never marry or have children; will have children who themselves are geriatric by the time that nursing facility admission becomes a pertinent subject for the parent; will have children who live at a considerable distance from them; or will outlive spouses and children while failing to execute advance directives while still decisionally capable. Additionally, in many cases, persons with severe mental problems, especially when accompanied by serious behavioral manifestations, begin their long-term care experience with family support but eventually "wear out" the patience—and hence the involvement—of relatives and friends who abandon them. Indeed, the absence of a satisfactory informal support system in the home is one of the most important risk factors for the need for nursing facility admission (Freedman, 1996).

Timely executed advance instruction and/or proxy directives may alleviate some of the decision making problems now encountered. No matter how much public and professional attention is devoted to this topic, though, the percentage of persons taking advantage of this opportunity will remain limited.

A significant percentage of future nursing facility admissions will be for short-term rehabilitative or subacute stays (e.g., following surgery), and many of these individuals will be capable of making all or most of their own decisions about medical and financial issues—if not immediately at the time of admission, then shortly thereafter. Many other future nursing facility residents, however, probably will be severely cognitively and/or emotionally impaired. As our ability to keep people away from permanent institutional placement as long as possible continues to improve, those who eventually are admitted for the remaining duration of their lives will have a much higher level of acuity than nursing facility residents did in earlier days. As residents live longer, with more chronic illnesses, more decisions requiring appropriate decision makers will need to be made over extended periods of time.

Initial decisions regarding nursing facility placement will need to be made and implemented increasingly within shortened periods of time, as cost-containment pressures continue to contract the process of discharge planning into a "whirlwind." The imperative for clear but creative public and institutional policies, procedures, and educational strategies that account for pertinent clinical, legal, ethical, and financial considerations represents a challenge that cannot be ignored.

ACKNOWLEDGMENTS

The research for this report was funded as part of a grant from the Ohio General Assembly, through the Ohio Board of Regents, to the Ohio Long-Term Care Research Project.

The author expresses appreciation to the numerous individuals who agreed to be interviewed for this research project; considerations of confidentiality preclude them from being specifically named here. Thanks, also, to the following individuals for their thoughtful comments on an earlier draft of this report: Robert Atchley, Jane Straker, Marissa Scala, Ronald Kozlowski, and Julia Nack. Larry Weiss, Ph.D., Scripps Gerontology Center of Miami University, provided helpful guidance as the project officer on this endeavor. All opinions and/or shortcomings, of course, are solely those of the author unless noted otherwise.

REFERENCES

Applebaum, P. S. (1990). Voluntary hospitalization and due process: The dilemma of *Zinermon v. Burch*. *Hospital and Community Psychiatry, 41*, 1059–1060.

Appelbaum, P. S. (1994). *Almost a revolution: Mental health law and the limits of change*. New York: Oxford University Press.

Barnes, A. P. (1992). Beyond guardianship reform: A reevaluation of autonomy and beneficence for a system of principled decision-making in long-term care. *Emory Law Journal, 41*, 633–760.

Barton, C. D., Jr., Millik, H. S., Orr, W. B., & Janofsky, J. S. (1996). Clinicians' judgment of capacity of nursing home patients to give informed consent. *Psychiatric Services, 47,* 956–960.

Bradley, E., Walker, L., Blechner, B., & Wetle, T. (1997). Assessing capacity to participate in discussions of advance directives in nursing homes: Findings from a study of the patient self-determination act. *Journal of the American Geriatrics Society, 45,* 79–83.

Brock, D. W. (1996). What is the moral authority of family members to act as surrogates for incompetent patients? *Milbank Quarterly, 74,* 599–618.

Brooke, V. (1991–1992). Meeting the challenge: Involuntary residents in the nursing home. *Journal of the Long-Term Care Administration, 19,* 9–14.

Burns, B. J., Wagner, H. R., Taube, J. E., Magaziner, J., Permutt, T., & Landerman, L. R. (1993). Mental health service use by the elderly in nursing homes. *American Journal of Public Health, 83,* 331–337.

Conrad, J. R. (1992). Granny dumping: The hospital's duty of care to patients who have nowhere to go. *Yale Law and Policy Review, 10,* 463–487.

Elon, R., & Pawlson, L. G. (1992). The impact of OBRA on medical practice within nursing facilities. *Journal of the American Geriatrics Society, 40,* 958–963.

Faden, R. R., & Beauchamp, T. L. (1986). *A history and theory of informed consent.* New York: Oxford University Press.

Fins, D. L. (1992). *Serving as guardian or conservator: A guide for agencies and individuals.* Worcester, MA: Jewish Family Services.

Freedman, V. A. (1996). Family structure and the risk of nursing home admission. *Journal of Gerontology: Social Sciences, 51B,* S61–S69.

Freeman, I. C. (1995). One more faulty solution is novelty without progress: A reply to "Medical decision-making for the unbefriended nursing home resident." *Journal of Ethics, Law, and Aging, 1,* 93–96.

Frolik, L. A., & Brown, M. C. (1992). *Advising the elderly or disabled client.* Englewood Cliffs, NJ: Rosenfeld Launer Publications.

Frolik, L. A., & Kaplan, R. L. (1995). *Elder law.* St. Paul, MN: West.

Gibson, J. M., & Nathanson, P. S. (1990 Suppl.). When someone else must decide: The New Mexico medical treatment guardianship program. *Generations, 14,* 43–46.

Gilbert, D. E. (1991). Increasing access to long-term care through Medicaid antidiscrimination laws. *Journal of Health and Hospital Law, 24,* 105–111, 135.

Gillick, M. R. (1995). Medical decision-making for the unbefriended nursing home resident. *Journal of Ethics, Law, and Aging, 1,* 87–92.

Gottlich, V. (1994). Protection for nursing facility residents under the ADA. *Generations, 18,* 43–47.

Herr, S. S., & Hopkins, B. L. (1994). Health care decision-making for persons with disabilities: An alternative to guardianship. *Journal of the American Medical Association, 271,* 1017–1022.

Hoffman, D. E., Boyle, P., & Levenson, S. A. (1995). *Handbook for nursing home ethics committees.* Washington, DC: American Association of Homes and Services for the Aging.

Iris, M. A. (1990 Suppl.). Threats to autonomy in guardianship decision making. *Generations, 14,* 39–41.

Kapp, M. B. (1994). Ethical aspects of guardianship. *Clinics in Geriatric Medicine, 10,* 501–512.

Kapp, M. B. (1995a). Medical decisionmaking for older adults in institutional settings: Is beneficence dead in an age of risk management? *Issues in Law and Medicine, 11,* 29–47.

Kapp, M. B. (1995b). Surrogate decision-making for the unbefriended: Social and ethical problem, legal solution? *Journal of Ethics, Law, and Aging, 1,* 83–85.

Kapp, M. B. (1997). Treating medical charts near the end of life: How legal anxieties inhibit good patient deaths. *University of Toledo Law Review, 28*(3), 521–546.

Kapp, M. B., & Mossman, D. (1996). Measuring decisional capacity: Cautions on the construction of a "capacimeter." *Psychology, Public Policy, and Law, 2,* 73–95.

Kazin, C. (1989). Nowhere to go and chose to stay: Using the tort of false imprisonment to redress involuntary confinement of the elderly in nursing homes and hospitals. *University of Pennsylvania Law Review, 137,* 903–927.

King, N. M. P. (1996). *Making sense of advance directives* (2nd ed.). Washington, DC: Georgetown University Press.

Kisor, A. J. (1996). Nursing facility admission agreements: An analysis of selected content. *Journal of Applied Gerontology, 15,* 294–313.

Knepper, K. (1996). Involuntary transfers and discharges of nursing home residents under federal and state law. *Journal of Legal Medicine, 17,* 215–275.

Komisar, H. L., Lambrew, J. M., & Feder, J. (1996). *Long-term care for the elderly: A chart book.* New York: Commonwealth Fund.

Lisi, L. B., Burns, A., & Lussenden, K. (1994). *National study of guardianship systems: Findings and recommendations.* Ann Arbor, MI: Center for Social Gerontology.

McCullough, L. B., & Wilson, N. L. (Eds.). (1995). *Long-term care decisions: Ethical and conceptual dimensions.* Baltimore: Johns Hopkins University Press.

Meier, D. E. (1997). Voiceless and vulnerable: Dementia patients without surrogates in an era of capitation. *Journal of the American Geriatrics Society, 45,* 375–377.

Meisel, A. (1995). Barriers to forgoing nutrition and hydration in nursing homes. *American Journal of Law and Medicine, 21,* 335–382.

Mezey, M., Mitty, E., Rappaport, M., & Ramsey, G. (1997). Implementation of the patient self-determination act (PSDA) in nursing homes in New York City. *Journal of the American Geriatrics Society, 45,* 43–49.

Miller, T. E., Coleman, C. H., & Cugliari, A. M. (1997). Treatment decisions for patients without surrogates: Rethinking policies for a vulnerable population. *Journal of the American Geriatrics Society, 45,* 369–374.

Molloy, D. W., Clarnette, R. M., Braun, E. A., Eisemann, M. R., & Sneiderman, B. (1991). Decision making in the incompetent elderly: The daughter from California syndrome. *Journal of the American Geriatrics Society, 39,* 396–399.

Moody, H. R. (1987). Ethical dilemmas in nursing home placement. *Generations, 11,* 16–23.

Murphy, P. T. (1996). Fighting for fairness: Keeping public wards in the community and out of nursing homes. *Elder Law Journal, 4,* 499–508.

Ouslander, J. G., & Osterweil, D. (1994). Physician evaluation and management of nursing home residents. *Annals of Internal Medicine, 120,* 584–592.

Pellegrino, E. D., & Thomasma, D. C. (1988). *For the patient's good: The restoration of beneficence in health care.* New York: Oxford University Press.

Rains v Belshe (1995). 32 Cal.App.4th 157, 38 Cal.Rptr.185 (Cal.App. 1 Dist.).

Reschovsky, J. D. (1996). Demand for and access to institutional long-term care: The role of Medicaid in nursing home markets. *Inquiry, 33,* 15–29.

Richards, E. P., III, & Rathbun, K. C. (1993). *Law and the physician: A practical guide*. Boston: Little, Brown.

Schmidt, W. C., Jr. (1995). *Guardianship: The court of last resort for the elderly and disabled*. Durham, NC: Carolina Academic Press.

Siemon, D., Balch, S., Hurme, S. B., & Sabatino, C. (1993). Public guardianship: Where is it and what does it need? *Clearinghouse Review, 27,* 588–599.

Smyer, M., Schaie, K. W., & Kapp, M. B. (Eds.). (1995). *Older adults' decision-making and the law*. New York: Springer Publishing Company.

Thomas, B. M. (1982). The rights of patients in nursing homes: When is there state action? *George Mason University Law Review, 5,* 315–337.

Wagner v Fair Acres Geriatric Center (1995 March 15). No. 94-1275 (3d Cir.).

Wetle, T. (Guest Ed.) (1995–1996). The nursing home revisited. *Generations, 19* [Special issue].

Whitton, L. S. (1996). Caring for the incapacitated: A case for nonprofit surrogate decision makers in the twenty-first century. *University of Cincinnati Law Review, 64,* 879–910.

Winick, B. J. (1994). How to handle voluntary hospitalization after *Zinermon* v. *Burch*. *Administration and Policy in Mental Health, 21,* 395–406.

Zimny, G. M., & Diamond, J. A. (1994). *Social service agencies as guardians of elderly wards: Final report*. St. Louis: Saint Louis University Health Sciences Center.

Zinermon v. Burch (1990). 494 U.S. 113.

Index

Acquired immunodeficiency syndrome, subacute care, 25
Activities of daily living, subacute care and, 28
Acute care
  alternatives to, impetus behind establishment of, 1
  long-term care, transition between, 1–22
ADL. See Activities of daily living
Adult day health care, 69–70
Adult Protective Services, role of, in nursing facility admission, 165
Advanced practice nurses, as providers of transitional care service, 8–9
Age, influence of, patient outcome and, 3
AIDS. See Acquired immunodeficiency syndrome
Alternatives to acute hospital care, impetus behind establishment of, 1
APNs. See Advanced practice nurses
Arizona, Medicaid, managed care, elderly, 138–139
Arthritis, subacute care, 28
Attending physicians, role in subacute care, 35
Auto accident, subacute care, 25

Berg functional balance test, geriatric day hospital, 82
Blood count, white, elevated, hospital readmission and, 3

Boston, Program for All Inclusive Care of Elderly model, 113
Britain, geriatric day hospital, 72–73
Bronx, Program for All Inclusive Care of Elderly model, 113

Capitation rates, Program for All Inclusive Care of Elderly model, 113t
CARE Program. See Collaborative Assessment and Rehabilitation for Elders program
Care sites, distance from, transitional service and, 8
Catheters, insertion of, in subacute care, 37
Chronic obstructive pulmonary disease, transitional care, 2
Clinical decision–making, factors influencing, 4–6
Clinical practice guidelines, managed care, elderly, 134–137
Coexisting conditions, subacute care and, 27
Cognitive status
  geriatric day hospital, 79–80
  hospital readmission and, 4
  referrals for transitional care services and, 5
Collaborative Assessment and Rehabilitation for Elders program, 77–78
  outcome measures, 78t

179

Columbia, Program for All Inclusive Care of Elderly model, 113
Commitment to nursing facility, 149–178
Communication among providers, effective discharge planning and, 7
Comorbidity
  functional dependency, subacute care and, 28–29
  subacute care and, 27, 27t
Congestive heart failure, subacute care, 25
Consent, to nursing facility admission, voluntariness issues, 149–178
Contusions, subacute care, 25
COPD. *See* Chronic obstructive pulmonary disease
Costs. *See also* Financing; Reimbursement
  factors relating to, 39t
  Medicare home health expansion, 112–115
  Program for All Inclusive Care of Elderly model, 112–115
  subacute care, 39t
  transitional care services, 6–9, 9
Culture
  nature of transitional care services used, 7–8
  in subacute care, 34t

DataPACE, 107–108
Denver, Program for All Inclusive Care of Elderly model, 113
Dependency, functional, subacute care and, 28–29
Depression, hospital readmission and, 4
Diabetes mellitus, hospital readmission and, 3
Discharge plans
  communication and, 7
  implementation of, 7
Distance from care sites, transitional service and, 8

Efficiency, subacute care and, 39
El Paso, Program for All Inclusive Care of Elderly model, 113

Elderly. *See* Geriatric day hospital; Program for All Inclusive Care of Elderly model
  managed care, 118–148
Emotional status, geriatric day hospital, 80–87
Endocarditis, subacute care, 25
Ethnicity, nature of transitional care services used, 7–8
Evaluation, of patient's functional ability, during hospitalization, 5

Falls, subacute care, 25
Financing, Program for All Inclusive Care of Elderly model, 104–105
Florida, Medicaid, managed care, elderly, 139
Fluids, administration of, in subacute care, 37
Fracture, hip, transitional care, 2
Functional dependency, subacute care and, 28–29
Functional independence measure, geriatric day hospital, 81–82
Functional status
  evaluation of, during hospitalization, 5
  geriatric day hospital, 81–83
    Berg functional balance test, 82
    functional independence measure, 81–82
    Tinetti Gait/balance assessment, 82–83
  hospital readmission and, 4
  referrals for transitional care services and, 5

Gastroenteritis, subacute care, 25
Gender, patient outcome and, 3
Geographic differences, in availability of services, 6
Geriatric day hospital, 67–87
  in Britain, 72–73
  clinical outcome measurement, 79–84
  cognitive status, 79–80

emotional status, 80–87
functional status, 81–83
  Berg functional balance test, 82
  functional independence measure, 81–82
  Tinetti Gait/balance assessment, 82–83
medical status, 79
nutritional status, 79
post discharge outcomes, 83
quality-of-life status, 81
sensory, and nutritional status, 79
sensory status, 79
Collaborative Assessment and Rehabilitation for Elders program, 77–78
outcome measures, 78t
community–based models, 68–71
  adult day care, 69
  adult day health care, 69–70
  geriatric day hospital, 71
  medical day care, 69–70
  partial hospital, 70–71
  senior center programs, 68–69
design, 75–76
evaluation, 74–77
research, 83–84
evolution of, 71–74
history of, 71–74
instrumentation, 76–77
patient population, 75
in United States, 73–74
Geriatricians, managed care, elderly, 132–134
Guardianship, nursing facility admission, voluntariness, 149–178

HCFA. *See* Health Care Financing Administration
Health Care Financing Administration
  clarification of Medicare statutory provisions, 46
  Medicare and Medicaid Statistical Supplement, 56–57
Health maintenance organization

managed care, elderly, 119, 128–131
  performance measurement systems, 122
  managed care, elderly, 122
  preferred provider organizations, 119
Health status, self-reported, hospital readmission and, 4
Heart disease, transitional care, 2
Heart failure
  congestive, subacute care, 25
  history of, hospital readmission with, 3
HEDIS. *See* Health maintenance organization performance measurement systems
Hip procedure, and hip fracture, transitional care, 2
Home care
  agency, hospitals with, 8
  managed care, elderly, 126–127
  Program for All Inclusive Care of Elderly model, 97
Hospital readmission, clinical variables predictive of, 3
Hospitalization prior to subacute stay, primary reasons for, 27t
Hypertension
  hospital readmission and, 3
  subacute care, 28

IEC. *See* Institutional ethics committee
Illness, subacute care, 24–26
  factors influencing outcomes of, 25–26
Inspector General, Office of, Medicare home health expansion, 56–57
Institutional ethics committee, role of, in nursing facility admission, 172
Insurance, influence, on transitional services, 8
Integrated financing, Program for All Inclusive Care of Elderly model, 104–105
Intensity, of transitional care services, 6–8
Interdisciplinary team, management, Program for All Inclusive Care of Elderly model, 98–105

Intermediate care units, hospitals with, transitional service and, 8
Interstate variation, Medicare home health care, 56–58

JCAHO. *See* Joint Commission on Accreditation of Healthcare Organizations
Joint Commission on Accreditation of Healthcare Organizations, 122–123

Left ventricular dysfunction, hospital readmission and, 4
Legal issues, consent, admission to nursing facility and, 149–178
Licensure, of subacute care, 36
Long-term care, acute care, transition between, 1–22
Lung abscess, complicating pneumonia, 27

Managed care
  elderly, 118–148
    acute, chronic care services, integration of, 127–140
    clinical practice guidelines, 134–137
    defined, 119
    enrollment, 120–122
    geriatricians, 132–134
    health maintenance organization, 128–131
      performance measurement systems, 122
    home health care, 126–127
    hospital use, 123–124
    Joint Commission on Accreditation of Healthcare Organizations, 122–123
    Medicaid, 137–140
    Medicare, screening, service coordination, 131–132
    multi-disciplinary teams, 132–134
    performance, 122–127
      monitoring of, 122–127
    physician use, 124–125
    procedures, 125–126
    provider participation, 120–122
    skilled nursing care, 126–127
    social organization, 128–131
    Tax Equity and Fiscal Responsibility Act, 120
    tests, 125–126
  subacute care and, 39
  subacute care reimbursement, 38
Medicaid
  managed care, elderly, 137–140
  private insurers, managed care, subacute care reimbursement, 38
Medical day care, geriatric care, 69–70
Medicare
  home health expansion, 45–66, 52
    expenditure growth, 49t
      causes of, 49–54
    future directions, 58–63
    growth rates, annual, 51
    home health benefit, evolution of, 46–49
    payments, 48t
    policy, 54–58
    research, 54–58
    utilization, 48t
  managed care, elderly, screening, service coordination, 131–132
  Prospective Payment System, alternatives to acute hospital care and, 1
  skilled nursing facility category, for providing post-acute care, 23
  subacute care reimbursement, 38
Medications, daily, hospital readmission and, 3
Minnesota, Medicaid, managed care, elderly, 139–140
Multidisciplinary team
  managed care, elderly, 132–134
  for promotion of transition, 9

National PACE Association, 111–112
NP. *See* Nurse practitioner

Index

Nurse practitioner, role in subacute care, 35–36
Nursing facility admissions, voluntariness, 149–178
Nutrients, administration of, in subacute care, 37
Nutritional services, Program for All Inclusive Care of Elderly model, 98
Nutritional status, geriatric day hospital, 79

Oakland, Program for All Inclusive Care of Elderly model, 113
Office of Inspector General, Medicare home health expansion, 56–57
OnLok model, history of, 89–91
Osteomyelitis, subacute care, 25
Outcomes, patient, factors related to, 3–4, 26t

PA. *See* Physician assistant
PACE model. *See* Program for All Inclusive Care of Elderly model
Partial hospital, geriatric care, 70–71
Patient outcome, factors related to, 3–4, 26t
Pelvic fracture, subacute care, 25
Perceived quality of life, hospital readmission and, 4
Petition, for guardianship, in nursing facility admission, 149–178, 162–164
Physician assistant, role in subacute care, 35–36
Physicians, role in care of subacute patients, 34–35
Plans, discharge, implementation of, 7
Pneumonia
 lung abscess complicating, 27
 subacute care, 25
Point of service plans, managed care, elderly, 119
Poisoning, subacute care, 25
Portland, Program for All Inclusive Care of Elderly model, 113

POS plan. *See* Point of service plan
PPO. *See* Preferred provider organization
PPS. *See* Prospective Payment System
Practitioner roles, subacute care, attributes, 34–36, 35t
Preferred provider organizations, managed care, elderly, 119
Primary care physician, role in subacute care, 35
Prior hospital admissions, hospital readmission and, 3
Private insurers, managed care, subacute care reimbursement, 38
Program for All Inclusive Care of Elderly model, 88–117
 acute, long-term care, integrated, 92–95
 acute medical problem
  flexibility, 103–104
  integrated financing, 104–105
  interdisciplinary team management, 98–105
 capitation rates 1996, 113t
 Community Health Accreditation Program, review by, 110
 cost, 112–115
 covered services, 93t
 current status of, 105–107
 DataPACE, 107–108
 description, 91–105
 evaluation studies, 109–110
 future directions, 115
 history of, 89–91
 inpatient utilization, cross–site comparison, 94t
 interdisciplinary team
  functions, 96–98
  home care, 97
  integrated care through, 95–96
  nursing, 96–97
  nutritional services, 98
  pharmacy, 97
  primary care, 96
  recreational therapy, 98
  rehabilitation, 97–98
  social work, 97
  transportation, 98

Program for All Inclusive Care *(cont.)*
  limitations of, 113–114
  National PACE Association, 111–112
  operational guidelines, 108
  protocol, 108–109
  quality assurance system, 110–111
  reimbursement, 112–115
  selection process, 91–92
  site, state-city, 113
Prospective Payment Commission, Medicare home health expansion, 56–57
Prospective payment system
  alternatives to acute hospital care and, 1
  for skilled nursing care, 40
Provider
  requirements, subacute care, 36–38
  transitional care services, 6–9
Psychotic individual, nursing facility admission, voluntariness, 151
Public guardianship systems, legislatively created, for nursing facility admission, 162–163

Quality assurance system, for Program for All Inclusive Care of Elderly model, 110–111
Quality of life
  as perceived, hospital readmission and, 4
  status, geriatric day hospital, 81

Race, nature of transitional care services used, 7–8
Radiation, subacute care, 25
Readmission, to hospital, clinical variables predictive of, 3
Recreational therapy, Program for All Inclusive Care of Elderly model, 98
Regulation, of subacute care, 36
Reimbursement
  Medicare home health expansion, 112–115

Program for All Inclusive Care of Elderly model, 112–115
  for subacute care, 38–41
Research-based models, transitional care, 9–10
  care management, 14–16
  day hospital, 10–11
  home health care, 11–13
    community nursing services, 12
    HMO follow-up services, 12
    hospital-based home care, 12
    integrated health systems, 14
    sub-acute care, 13–14
Respiratory infections, subacute care, 25
Rheumatoid arthritis, subacute care, 28
Rochester, Program for All Inclusive Care of Elderly model, 113

Sacramento, Program for All Inclusive Care of Elderly model, 113
San Francisco, Program for All Inclusive Care of Elderly model, 113
Self-reported health status, hospital readmission and, 4
Senior center programs, 68–69
Serum sodium levels, abnormal, hospital readmission and, 3
Severity of illness, subacute care and, 28–29
Skilled nursing care
  managed care, elderly, 126–127
  prospective payment system for, 40
Skilled nursing facility, category, for providing post-acute care, 23
Social support, hospital readmission and, 4
Sociodemographic characteristics, access to transitional care services and, 6
Specialists, role in subacute care, 35
Sprains, subacute care, 25
Stroke
  subacute care, 25
  transitional care, 2
Subacute care, 23–44

assessment, 33
care goals, objectives, 33
characterization of, 26–29
clinical programs, 30–31
comorbidities, 27t
costs of care, 39t
cultures, relevant, features of, 34t
defined, 29–30
essential processes of, 33t
factors promoting growth of, 23–24
follow-up, 33
future needs, 41
hospitalization, prior to subacute stay, primary reasons for, 27t
iatrogenic problems, prevention of, 33
illness, 24–26
  factors influencing outcomes of, 25–26
  as interdisciplinary undertaking, 31–36
licensure, 36
managed care and, 39
nosocomial problems, prevention of, 33
participants in, 31
patient selection, 33
planning, 33
post-selection/preadmission, 33
practitioner roles, attributes, 34–36, 35t
procedures, 37t
processes of, 33t
programs, 30t
provider requirements, 36–38
regulation, 36
reimbursement, 38–41
settings for health care delivery, shifts in, 24
team approach, 31–34
treatments, 37t
Surrogate decisionmaking, judicially appointed, in nursing facility admissions, 162
Swing beds, hospitals with, transitional service and, 8

Tax Equity and Fiscal Responsibility Act, managed care, elderly, 120

Team. *See also* Interdisciplinary team
  management, Program for All Inclusive Care of Elderly model, 98–105
  managed care, elderly, 132–134
  multidisciplinary, for promotion of transition, 9
  Program for All Inclusive Care of Elderly model, 98–105
  subacute care, 31–34
TEFRA. *See* Tax Equity and Fiscal Responsibility Act
Tinetti Gait/balance assessment, geriatric day hospital, 82–83
Transitional care
  costs for, 9
  defined, 1
  intensity of, 6–8
  models of, 9–10
  patients in need of, 2–6
  providers of, 8–9
  settings, 1–15
Tubes, insertion of, in subacute care, 37

Upper respiratory infections, subacute care, 25
U.S. General Accounting Office, Medicare home health expansiion, 56–57

Ventilatory failure, subacute care, 25
Ventricular dysfunction, hospital readmission and, 4
Viral gastroenteritis, subacute care, 25
Voluntariness, nursing facility admissions, 149–178

White blood count, elevated, hospital readmission and, 3
Wisconsin
  Medicaid, managed care, elderly, 139
  Program for All Inclusive Care of Elderly model, 113

Zinermon v. Burch, nursing facility admission, consent issues, 152

Springer Publishing Company

Assisted Living Administration
The Knowledge Base

James E. Allen, PhD, MSPH

In recent years, assisted living facilities have begun to dominate the field of nursing home administration. These facilities serve the health care market segment of persons who are no longer are able to live independently and need help with the activities of daily living but not 24-hour nursing care.

In this cutting edge text, James Allen introduces the reader to this new and growing industry. He explores the newly established domains of practice which include organizational management; human resources management; business and financial considerations; laws surrounding physical environment; and resident care.

This volume is intended as a text for professionals in certification training, as well as a resource for the seasoned administrator.

Contents: Foreword • Acknowledgments • Introduction

Part I: Assisted Living Industry Overview Management, Leadership

Part II: Assisted Living Facility Organizational Patterns; Human Resources

Part III: Assisted Living Facility Financing, Business Operations

Part IV: The Assisted Living Facility Environment: The Long Term Care Continuum Laws and Regulations

Part V: Assisted Living Facility Resident Care

Final Observations • Appendix A • Appendix B

1999   640pp (est.)   0-8261-1253-6   *hardcover*

536 Broadway, New York, NY 10012-3955 • (212) 431-4370 • Fax (212) 941-7842

Ⓢ *Springer Publishing Company*

Assessing Satisfaction in Health and Long-Term Care
Practical Approaches to Hearing the Voices of Consumers
Robert Applebaum, MSW, PhD
Jane Straker, PhD, and **Scott Geron,** PhD

Emphasizing how consumer satisfaction data can be used as part of an overall quality improvement approach for health and long-term care services, this book provides practical advice on such issues as concepts, and measures; data collection approaches and sampling; and analysis and interpretation of satisfaction results. Of interest to both practitioners and researchers.

Partial Contents: Part I. Examining Consumer Satisfaction: Context and Methods • Why the Growing Interest in Consumer Satisfaction? • Part II. Approaches to Measuring Consumer Satisfaction • Measuring Consumer Satisfaction in Home Care

1999   224pp (est.)   0-8261-1262-5   *hardcover*

Satisfaction Surveys in Long-Term Care
Editors: **Jiska Cohen-Mansfield,** PhD
Farida Ejaz, PhD, and **Perla Werner,** PhD

LTC facilities, like all service providers, need to measure client satisfaction and recruit information as a part of everyday business. The authors show how to convert various kinds of feedback from LTC clients into useable measures of business performance. Includes an array of surveys and scales to assess and improve the quality of care services.

1999   224pp (est.)   0-8261-1289-6

Springer Publishing Company

New Ways to Care for Older People
Building Systems Based on Evidence
Evan Calkins, MD, **Chad Boult**, MD, MPH
Edward H. Wagner, MD, MPH, **James T. Pacala**, MD, MS

The editors systematically examine successful interventions and those which fail to improve health outcomes among the full range of older people – from triathletes to those near the end of life. Focusing primarily on the person, rather than on the facilities or professionals providing care, the editors describe optimal systems of care. This book is a valuable reference for all health service administrators, medical directors, health providers, researchers, and policy makers concerned with the design and evaluation of improved systems of health.

Contents: Preface, *T.F. Williams* • Foreword, *R.L. Kane*
Section I. When the Older Person is Healthy and Independent • Prevention of Frailty, *D.M. Buchner* • Prevention of Disease, *J.T. Pacala*
Section II. When the Older Person is Chronically Ill or at Risk • Care of Older People with Chronic Illness, *E.H. Wagner* • Care of Older People at Risk, *C. Boult*
Section III. When the Older Person is Acutely Ill • Care of Acute Illness in the Home, *B. Leff and J.R. Burton* • Emergency Care, *C.J. Michalakes et al.* • Care of Older People in the Hospital, *E. Calkins and B.J. Naughton* • Subacute Care, *T. von Sternberg et al.* • Rehabilitation, *A.M. Kramer* • Care of Older People Who are Dying, *R.M. McCann*
Section IV. When the Older Person is Disabled • Overview of Community-Based Long-Term Care, *A.B. Ford* • Community-Based Long-Term Care, *W.G. Weissert and S.C. Hedrick* • Comprehensive Care of People with Alzheimer's Disease, *D. Johnston and B.V. Reifler* • Long-Term Care in the Nursing Home, *D.B. Reuben and J.F. Schnelle*
Section V. Concluding Observations • Integrating Quality Assurance Across Sites of Care, *E.A. Coleman and R.W. Besdine* • Integrating Care, *C. Boult and J.T. Pacala* • The Role of the Older Person in Managing Illness, *M. Von Korff and E.H. Wagner* • Medicare and Managed Care, *H.S. Luft* • Necessary Changes in the Infrastructure of Health Systems, *G. Halvorson*

1998   280pp   0-8261-1220-X   *hardcover*

536 Broadway, New York, NY 10012-3955 • (212) 431-4370 • Fax (212) 941-7842

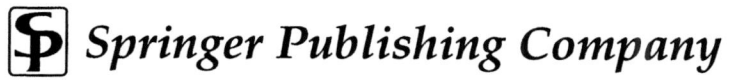 *Springer Publishing Company*

Restraint-Free Care
A Guide for Individualized Clinical Practice
Neville E. Strumpf, PhD, RN, C, FAAN
Joanne E. Patterson, PhD, RN
Joan Stockman Wagner, MSN, CRNP
Lois K. Evans, DNSc, RN, FAAN

This book is for individuals seeking information on restraint-free care. Organized in outline format, the authors highlight critical material to be readily adaptable as a quick reference for clinicians, or as an adjunct for teaching staff or educating administrators, board members, and consumers.

A philosophy of individualized care is the framework for this guide, which the authors believe to be the key to understanding older adults and to providing restraint-free care. The goals of individualized care include promoting comfort and safety, optimizing function and independence, and achieving the greatest possible quality of life. Such care requires clinicians to make sense of behavior rather than to control responses of clients.

The book contains specific strategies of understanding behavior; effecting change for the individual, the environment and institution; managing the risk of falls; and interference with recent treatments. Case studies and lists of resources are included in this practical and information-packed resource.

Contents:

Preface • Rethinking Restraint Use • Implementing a Process of Change • Making Sense of Behavior • Responding to Behavioral Phenomena • Assessment and Prevention of Falls and Injurious Falls • Caring for the Person Who Interferes with Treatment • Maintaining a Process of Change

1998   168pp   0-8261-1215-3   softcover

536 Broadway, New York, NY 10012-3955 • (212) 431-4370 • Fax (212) 941-7842

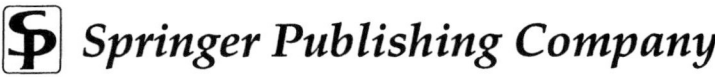 **Springer Publishing Company**

Risk Management in Long-Term Care
A Quick Reference Guide
Andrew Weinberg, MD, FACP

"Risk Management and Long Term Care is full of case examples, specific suggestions and recommended policies and procedures to follow in providing quality care and thereby managing risk."
—from the foreword by James L. Wilkes, II, Esq.

A practical, effective, and thorough risk management tool, this book helps health professionals address common problem areas in order to avoid litigation. Potential risk topics covered include: injury from physical restraint, resident abuse and neglect, infection control, polypharmacy and medication use, and much more. The volume also features valuable information on how to respond to legal claims. Each chapter concludes with 10 tips for the reader. The appendices contain case studies with questions for discussion and a useful resource list of organizations. This handy guide is indispensable to administrators, nurses, and physicians, as well as students of health administration.

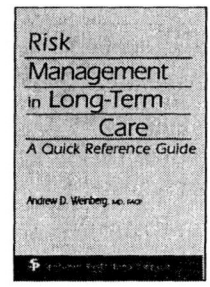

> **Contents:** Introduction and Overview • Approach to Risk Management in the Long-Term Care Setting • Pressure Ulcers • Issues Related to Polypharmacy and Medication Use • Physical Restraints and Neuropsychoactive Medication Use • Infection Control Issues • Prevention of Resident Neglect or Abuse • Falls and Resident Safety Concerns • The Role of the Medical Director • Legal Aspects of Risk Management • Creating and Implementing an Effective Risk Management Program • Risk Management in the 1990s and Beyond • Case Presentations and Question Review
>
> 1997   128pp   0-8261-9940-2   *hardcover*

536 Broadway, New York, NY 10012-3955 • (212) 431-4370 • Fax (212) 941-7842